HEALTHCARE CRISIS 2025: A Clinical Perspective

By

J Smith

About the Author

Jean Smith is a highly accomplished healthcare executive, certified by the American College of Healthcare Executives. With an MBA focused on Leadership, she has a proven track record of elevating healthcare teams to achieve the next level of excellence. Jean combines her extensive knowledge of healthcare and various industries with leadership coaching to drive meaningful change and improvement.

Her expertise includes creating a profitable for-profit business through a hospital joint venture, as well as authoring the successful application leading a multi-hospital system to triumph in the prestigious Baldrige Journey, the highest state-level award for quality. Additionally, she has served as a Baldrige Examiner at the national level.

With experience in both permanent and interim leadership roles across 13 states, Jean's mission remains clear: to improve the quality of patient-centered care and help healthcare organizations reach their full potential.

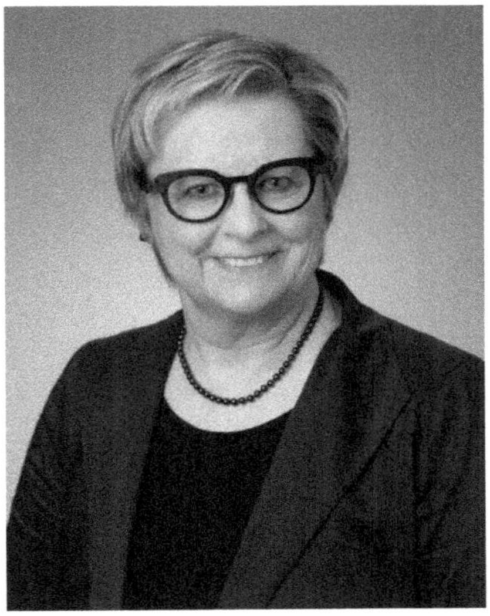

Table of Contents

FIGURES

GLOSSARY (* denotes billing definitions)

Accreditation — self assessment and external peer assessment process used to assess excellence with established standards and to continuously improve.

Affordable Care Act/Obamacare (ACA) — comprehensive health care reform law passed in 2010 during the Obama administration. The goals were: make health insurance coverage more affordable, expand Medicaid where possible, and support innovation to lower health care costs.

AHEAD — All Payor Health Equity Approaches and Development Model- Three cohorts of selected hospitals for participation in a CMS incentive program, to advance the primary care coordination model; to roll out in January 2026 and January 2027.

AHRQ — Department of Health & Human Services, Agency for Healthcare Research- Mission to improve healthcare for all by producing evidence to make healthcare of higher quality, making it safer, patient-centered, timely, effective, accessible, efficiently provided, and equitably distributed.

Baldrige Performance Excellence Program — National quality Presidential award with standards for proven leadership and management practices for high performance; State excellence programs also utilize the same standards; after an exhaustive evaluation of a detailed application showing sustained results, winners are chosen annually for this award, considered the highest-level award in quality.

Beckers Healthcare — the "go to" digital information newsletter reporting on the most critical issues in American healthcare with current and past data provided.

CareCompare — the name of a streamlined redesign of eight Center for Medicare & Medicaid Services (CMS) healthcare comparison tools available on Medicare.gov launched during the previous Trump administration; provides information for informed decisions about healthcare based on cost, quality of care, volume of services and other data. www.medicare.gov/care-compare.

Capitalism — an economic system characterized by private or corporate ownership of capital goods, by investments that are determined by private decision, and by prices, production, and the distribution of goods that are determined mainly by competition in a free market.

Center for Medicare (1965) & Medicaid Service (CMS) — a Federal agency providing health coverage through Medicare, Medicaid, Children's Health Insurance Program and the Health Insurance Marketplace; partners with the entire health care community to improve quality, equity, and outcomes.

Communism — branch of *socialism* similar in that it's still founded on the idea of collective cooperation but differs in that communists believe that cooperation should be run by a totalitarian government made up of one and *only one* government.

***Cost reimbursement** — payment is based on what has happened in the past and allowable costs are created based on the cost of care; coverages are defined in policy; Critical Access hospitals are paid on cost reimbursement while larger hospitals have been switched to fee-for-service and DRGs.

C-Suite — the name for the group of chiefs employed by a hospital or system, making up the main leadership; depending on size and volume, may consist of Chief Nursing Officer (CNO), Chief Financial Officer (CFO), Chief Operating Officer (COO), Chief Medical Officer (CMO), Chief Quality Officer (CQO) and Chief Executive Officer (CEO) at the highest level. Often, the Vice President of Quality (VPQ) is part of the decision-making team.

Democracy — a form of government in which the supreme power is vested in the people and exercised directly by them or by their elected agents under a free electoral system. Capitalism is part of Democracies.

***Diagnostic Related Groups (DRG)** — Medicare utilizes set fees for 518 specific diagnoses and was nationally launched in 1983 during the Reagan administration to control spiraling healthcare costs; a hospital must watch costs to make a profit or lose Medicare dollars in reimbursement.

Electronic Medical Record (EHR) — an individual electronic medical record utilized by providers to store health information in a digital format versus a paper chart, with the intent of providing efficiencies.

Failure Mode Effects Analysis (FMEA) — quality improvement tool initially established in 1949 by the military and NASA; systematic approach to proactively design or improve an existing process by identifying possible failures, causes, effects and how to mitigate them or prevent them.

***Fee-for-Service** — traditional payment model for reimbursement to providers for each service delivered to a patient; utilizes ICD-10 Coding to bill, which is very itemized and detailed.

Gross Domestic Product (GDP) — total value of goods and services produced and sold on the market in a country in a given period; serves as a gauge of our economy's overall size and health; percent afforded to healthcare services utilized to compare expenditures globally. (Figure 1A/1B, Pages 9/10)

German Federal Ministry of Health — central tasks include safeguarding and advancing efficiency of statutory health insurance and long-term care insurance systems, strengthening patients' interests and ensuring cost-effectiveness and affordability of the healthcare system.

***Global capitation** — a provider or organization is paid a fixed monthly payment for each enrolled patient; covers all services so incentivizes cost control; utilized in population healthcare.

Institute for Healthcare Improvement (IHI) — Established in 1991, is a *globally* recognized not-for-profit health care improvement organization, applying evidence-based methods to meet current and future challenges; provides tools and resources along with consulting services.

Institute of Medicine (IOM) — an independent, not-for-profit organization working outside of government to provide unbiased, authoritative advice to decision makers; established in the 1960s because of politicized debates on national health insurance during the Kennedy and Johnson administrations.

ISO9000 Series of Standards — published by the International Organization for Standardization (ISO) which is composed of more than 160 countries to assist companies in satisfying customers, meet regulatory requirements, and achieve continual improvement; provides accreditation for many industries, starting in 1987.

Medication Reconciliation — process of comparing new medication orders to all medications patient has been taking to avoid medication errors; this is especially labor intensive with high numbers of medications and EHR software does not support this safety need currently.

Medicare Payment Advisory Commission (MEDPAC) — an independent, Congressional legislative branch agency in Washington, DC, formulating policy issues for Congressional recommendation, including payments; reports are issued in March and June each year-budget request 2025 is 14.5m, an increase of 4.7% from 2024.

National Association for Healthcare Quality (NAHQ) — a private organization formed in 1976 providing healthcare quality professionals resources for education, certification, and competency; goal is to reduce variability in care delivery and drive value through improved quality and safety outcomes.

National Quality Foundation (NQF) — Federal organization structured as a public-private collaborative; mission to promote delivery of high-quality health care and is relied upon by the Federal government for defining measures or practices as best, evidence-based approaches to improving care.

Pharmacy Benefit Manager (PBM) — third parties that go between health insurance providers and drug manufacturers to negotiate costs and payments; also create formularies (which prescription drugs best to utilize).

Population Healthcare — based on primary care provider management, care coordination is improved and supported by appropriate financial and care models; this includes contracting and partnering with multiple players to cover services at a negotiated fee (may use the global capitation model).

Principle of Solidarity — a socio-ethical and political concept which states that it is fair; benefits and obligations are justly shared between members of the society, and *those most vulnerable and in need receive preferential concern* (Catholic bishop addition). A theory or system of social organization that advocates the vesting of ownership and control of the means of production and distribution, of capital, land, etc., in the community as a whole.

***Professional Fees** — separate billing in a hospital stay to cover providers only; reimbursement is in addition to facility fees.

Promoting Interoperability Programs/Meaningful use — incentivizes and penalizes hospitals for whether they meet criteria showing they promote Federal objectives to create a future where shared information is possible; premise is this would reduce negative outcomes associated with fragmented care and assist workflows with improved communications.

Revenue Cycle Management — process named to manage and staff all financial operations from initial patient appointment, insurance verifications, through billing, collecting, and handling denials.

Root Cause Analysis — performance improvement structured method, reactive in nature, to analyze adverse events after they occur, and problem solve to prevent future events.

Socialism — economic and political theories or movements advocating collective or governmental ownership and administration of the means of production with equal distribution of goods.

The Joint Commission (TJC) — accredits hospitals and provides specialty certifications with rigorous, researched standards to promote a "Gold Seal of Approval" for safety and quality; independent, not-for-profit company; CMS must approve TJC and competitors to provide hospital approval on their behalf (deemed authority).

***Value-based Care or Purchasing (VBP)** — a newer approach than fee-for-service service rendered; CMS and other payors individually create quality incentive programs with varying metrics based on maximizing reimbursement.

INTRODUCTION

I was taught when you have passion for a mission, you must answer the call. My father passed away at 52 years of age when I was 13. It was the 1960's and, looking at the capabilities and equipment in healthcare today, it was very backward. I made a promise to relieve suffering in healthcare as I am able and improve the quality of care wherever I may land. I recently retired from hospital administration after 50 years as a Registered Nurse. The opportunities received over those years are amazing. An MBA allowed me to experience the C-Suite Leadership Team as a Chief Nursing Officer a few times, then resonating as a leader in Quality, working in 14 hospitals in 13 states. One hospital hired me to start an equipment business, where I learned how to write a business plan, how to change management styles as a business grows, and how to ensure revenue exceeds expenses. And setting up a computer software system for billing and inventory—quite the task at the same time—helping me develop gratitude for folks in Information Systems departments!

As a cancer survivor of 13 years, I experienced healthcare as a satisfied patient. Living in Texas, I received the best local care possible at a most vulnerable time. That should be everyone's experience.

So, join me in evaluating healthcare today, both the good and challenging parts, and how this complex industry might better be understood, allowing leaders at every level to ensure America provides the safest, patient-centered healthcare where we live.

In Part 1, the Health Reform Security Act of 1998, proposed but not passed, is utilized to globally analyze what various parts of change were carried forward and what was not, as well as what we know as of 2024.

Part 2 proceeds to break down major areas of challenge and what is needed now while closing the loop on the Health Security Act discussion.

Part 3 combines a future vision of higher reliability, the Hedgehog Concept (*Good to Great*), and the Baldrige Performance Excellence standards to stimulate discussion about what can be done in the various stakeholder venues to get us there.

It is the intent of this book to demonstrate the need for expediency of change today in healthcare and how that can only be accomplished quickly and efficiently at the State and local levels, with more collaboration.

"The politicians debated how to *fund* health care, but what we really need to talk about is how to *fix* health care."

Marty Makary, MD, The Johns Hopkins Hospital, author of *The Price We Pay.*

PART 1

THEN & NOW: 1998 & 2024

Chapter 1

NON-PARTISAN HISTORY OF AN AMERICAN PROBLEM

Former President Bill Clinton served from 1993-2000 in the Oval Office. Although our political philosophies diverged, he impressed me in many ways: First, he commanded an audience to listen, inspiring trust; Second, he was brave to tackle the problems in healthcare; Third, he assigned Hillary to research and recommend healthcare reforms, based on evidence from the people working in healthcare. The topic of healthcare reform is generally avoided because it is emotional and difficult.

James Morone, a professor of political science who studied health care policy through the presidents, says the idea of government helping people buy private insurance evolved from its initiation with George H. Bush, through Clinton, George W. Bush, then Obama, who implemented it as Obamacare. George H.'s team of advisers left a very powerful legacy, figuring out ways to have government-enhanced private markets rather than simply create government programs in the Great Society model. George H. Bush refined what Nixon did to some extent! [1] What we now know as Obamacare (2010) has actually been bipartisan, evolving over the years.

In 1993, the Clintons put together the Health Security Act and published the book, "*Health Security: The President's Report to the American People*". [2] The balance of the discussion here will paraphrase and compare then to now— the official text fills in details very well if you wish to delve further. This proposal did not pass the budget that year, being late to the game, but the plan is well-researched and documented, lending us a springboard for innovation of great value.

At about the same time of this publication, I entered the Michigan State University Executive MBA Program, housed near Detroit. As the center of the automotive industry, teammates included those employed by the "Big Three" automobile companies—Ford, General Motors, and Chrysler. They were passionate about higher healthcare costs per vehicle threatening profitability. Higher insurance costs per employee, which they provide as a benefit, translate into increased costs they may or may not recover in revenue. Their question: why can't healthcare handle cost control when there are so many intelligent people in the industry? So, the battle of the minds began.

---

[1] Newman, K. (2018, December 5). The health care legacy of George H.W. Bush. *U.S. News & World Report.* https://www.usnews.com

[2] Clinton, B., & Clinton, H. R. (1993). *Health security: The president's report to the American people.* Touchstone Book.

Naively, I suggested one of our first projects should be the business of healthcare. The learning was swift and painful—they thought we were simply poor managers. Oh, that it could be that simple. I set out to increase their knowledge in the short time we had to do our project. I actually hoped to hear whether they might offer innovative ideas from a different perspective to balance cost, quality, and access to excellent care. As a young student, I failed that experiment. However, the experience drove me to find out more. I needed more experience and understanding to communicate healthcare's complexity and prove to them that failing to reduce costs was <u>not</u> simply due to business incompetence.

Thankfully, during my research, *"Leading Transformational Change"*[3] was published in 2001 by the American College of Healthcare Executives. Utilizing a business perspective, a physician internist partnered with a human resource executive, reconciling the business aspects of healthcare with the values at the heart of medicine. They laid out cultural factors focusing on occupational differences and *conflicting agendas*. This means that physicians, CEOs, CNOs, CMOs, CFOs, Unions, Payors, and other staff have colliding goals—built into the fabric of their specific occupations. The concept that changed my thinking completely was their comparison of the <u>Expert</u> culture to the <u>Collective</u> culture.

To summarize, the Expert culture (generally exemplified by the physician group) does not need Mission statements (business model) to strive for excellence and are characterized by individualized behavior. They do not seek teaming in the same way as Collectives, where affiliation is the major motivational experience. The authors state that, for the most part, other clinicians are Collectives. These are general statements but resonate with merit while observing a hospital interdisciplinary team striving to improve care. It is interesting, as well, to note the authors believe "The reasons people are attracted to collective or expert cultures are found in their respective socialization experiences." There are no villains.

Bottom line: the contentious nature of healthcare is either caused or exacerbated by diverse groups pushing various agendas while reaching for the same goal in excellence. Teaming is very much appreciated when all perspectives come together for a better solution (business concept). Independent thinking is appreciated when a surgeon is performing surgery on anyone. How can we possibly bridge this cultural gulf? It's like a marriage of opposites! Combined with the high turnover and mobility of strategic leaders, a high degree of difficulty and instability emerges. The authors present the need for partnerships to succeed with the Expert culture.

---

[3] Atchison, T. A., & Bujak, J. S. (2001). *Leading transformational change: The physician-executive partnership.* Health Administration Press.

There is more to say about how important culture is for the future because, as we are taught in basic business, culture eats strategy for breakfast (Peter Drucker). For now, back to history.

The Clinton Health Security Act (1993) is based on 6 Basic Principles, with more detail in the following chapters:

1. Security- Universal Healthcare
2. Simplicity- less paperwork
3. Savings- buying clout for small and large businesses
4. Quality- preventative care
5. Choice- right to choose
6. Responsibility- every employer with employee contribution

Where are we 31 years later? Let's start here to paraphrase and compare with some Takeaways along the way.

Chapter 1 TAKEAWAYS

1. Let's talk "FIX" along with "FUND"
2. Government-enhanced private markets leading to Obamacare evolved from the 1960's to 2010
3. Clinton's 1993 Health Security Act focuses on more innovation
4. Healthcare is a complex business with cultural challenges mainly built into the variety of providers
5. This discussion utilizes the Clinton recommendations of 1993 as a foundation of discussion in 2024

Chapter 2

SECURITY- Guaranteeing comprehensive benefits to all Americans

Health Security Act- limits healthcare premium increases, sets maximum out-of-pocket expense, more coverage for prescriptions, and expands access.

On benefits for All: The Gross Domestic Product (GDP) percentage as a total value of goods and services produced in a country for a given period is a metric used to indicate improvement and benchmarking (Figure 1A, Page 9). This graph depicts differences in the United States (U.S.) and other major countries.[4] Note the United States has the highest contribution at the end of 2022, even with the recent drop during the Pandemic.

Universal Healthcare, or healthcare for all, brought forward by the Clintons, is very debatable, with definition and implementation varying across countries and political beliefs. Refer to the Glossary for specific definitions of different economic systems, including capitalism, communism, principle of solidarity and socialism, often utilized in debating the issue. Guaranteeing benefits to all is beyond the scope of this publication and will not be argued here, however, questions might include: 1) Do other countries have less cost and higher taxes while caring for all? And 2) Do quality outcomes actually exceed the United States and, 3) how is this measured to assure the ability to compare reasonably?

Michael Chernew, Department of Health Care Policy, Harvard University, was asked whether costs would go down with benefits for all. His answer is no, if not combined with reducing low-value items.[5] He has performed studies of different benefit designs and is currently Chair of the Medicare Payment Advisory Commission (MedPAC).

German Model: In comparing American customer demands (low wait times, choice, coverage for pre-existing conditions) to others in the list, the German model seems to match the U.S. best. Figure 1A shows an 11.8% total contribution of healthcare dollars (GDP in 2022) for Germany. The United States, for the same time, was 16.5% (dropped due to the Pandemic), rose to 17.6% for 2023, returning to pre-Pandemic levels, and projected to reach 19.7% by 2032.[6] This begs the question: Could a hybrid American model, if constructed well, decrease costs and preserve choice? Although Germany's external cultural philosophies are vastly different than ours, which may provide

---

[4] **Statista.** (2024). Healthcare spending statistics. *Statista.* https://www.statista.com

[5] Harvard Online. (2024, February 12). *U.S. healthcare spending: Myths, facts, & strategies.* Webinar by Leemore Dafny & Michael Chernew.

[6] Health Affairs. (2024). National health expenditure projections, 2023-32. *Health Affairs, 43*(7), 910-921.

insurmountable challenges in the U.S., it is worth investigation to determine what might be possible.

Figure 1A HEALTHCARE EXPENDITURES

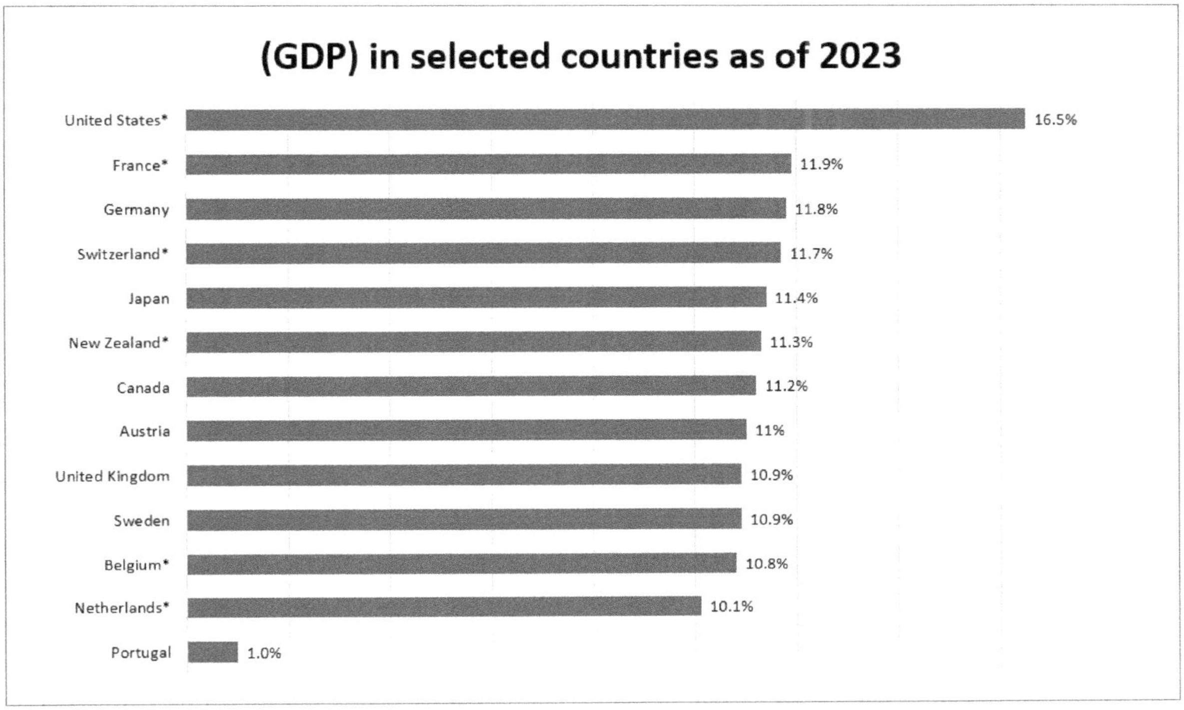

Germany, the most comparable in design, is 4.7% lower. Why?

In 2000 US GDP was **13.2%**, 2021 was **18.3%**, 2023 was **17.6%.** The **Health Security Act** projected **19%** by 2000. Now 19.7% is projected by 2032 per Health Affairs, July 2024

The rationale for the heavy decrease in 2020 while increasing each year: U.S. economy shrank by 3.5 percent in 2020 as the **coronavirus pandemic** ravaged factories, businesses and households, pushing U.S. economic growth to a low not seen since the United States wound down wartime spending in 1946. Also, medical services were down as were the use of medical supplies, and drugs as deaths increased.

Current health expenditure (% of GDP) | Data (worldbank.org)

FIGURE 1B

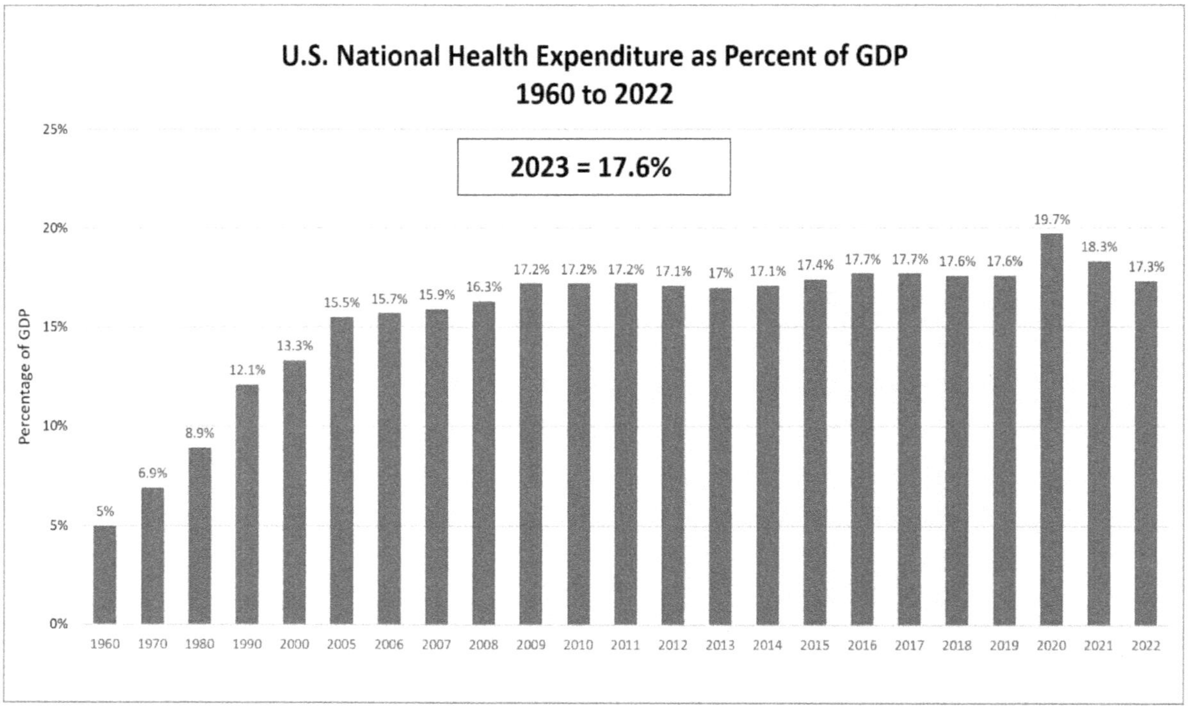

Visiting Germany and studying their healthcare program, the University of Michigan Public Health Students[7] found these major differences:

1. Pharmaceutical occupations are more tightly regulated
2. Nurses are not specialized and become registered after a 7-month curriculum in Germany
3. There is a solidarity concept—young pay for the old; rich pay for the poor; healthy pay for the sick; singles pay for families—held as a cultural value.

Also included in this ***Principle of Solidarity***—is a multi-payor system—statutory insurance for those with less of a certain salary, private insurance for more earnings, which includes more choice; employers/employees pay for most of the costs through premiums—all workers contribute about 7.5% salary into a public health insurance pool. Employers match that 7.5% contribution.[8]

Pharmacy - For the top three German program differences, the Michigan students noted U.S. pharmaceutical regulation is being pursued as a priority in the U.S. There is action afoot with the government and the private sector to better manage pharmaceutical costs, capping certain types of drugs and strict limits on out-of-pocket expenses

[7] Michigan School of Public Health. (2018, April 18). *Comparing the German and American healthcare systems.* University of Michigan. https://sph.umich.edu

[8] Edwards, J., & Dunn, J. (2019, June 30). Is Germany's health care system a model for the U.S.? *NBC News.* https://www.nbcnews.com

(Inflation Care Reduction Act, August 2022). In January 2022, Mark Cuban, a private entrepreneur, opened an online pharmacy, Cost Plus, to remove the middleman and reduce the costs of Pharmacy Benefit Management (PBM) companies. He claimed this could easily save millions of dollars. Other start-ups are following, but also leaders are realizing there are patient care advantages of PBM. For example, 1) claims in one pool allowing safety checks which prevent overuse, 2) lack of proper coordination for dangers of medication interaction, 3) possible reduction of opportunities for customers in defraying costs when medications are not covered.

Insulin out-of-pocket expense was regulated in the Biden administration. This is a chronic, high-risk disease with negative health implications over time if not treated and is the eighth cause of death in the United States. Also, based on projections of diabetic increase in younger patients, selecting this as a focus is of great value for a community's quality of life.

Nurses - There is a HUGE difference between German philosophy and the influence of bedside nurses and staff in assuring patient safety. There are many studies providing evidence of this. For example, one study in January 2022 concluded, "Nurses with positive safety attitudes reported fewer patient falls, medication errors, pressure injuries, healthcare-associated infections, mortality, physical restraints, vascular access device reactions, and higher patient satisfaction. Effective teamwork led to a reduction in adverse patient outcomes."[9] Although there are generally no differences in pay for our nursing education up to the Master's level—associate or bachelor's degrees—the push toward educational development and competency shows the American strategy for safer care is important. In the U.S., nurses can become physician extenders as Physician Assistants (PA) and Advanced Nurse Practitioners, providing avenues for advancement. Higher education is encouraged and tuition is a standard hospital benefit. The Magnet Program, a nursing excellence program, outlines higher levels of education for bedside nurse leaders and quality indicators they call "nurse-sensitive", defining further cause-and-effect outcomes for which nursing is personally held accountable and make an essential difference.

Another major difference is <u>*physician salaries*</u>, which are much lower in Germany than in the U.S. and based on a prospective free-for-service basis with global capitation. Each year, the German government sets the budget for health expenditures, and the money apportioned among health insurers and providers regionally. If utilization is higher, provider payments <u>are lowered proportionally</u>![10] *Tough sell in American business.*

---

[9] Nurse Open. (2022, January). Systematic review: Nurses' safety attitudes and their impact on patient outcomes in acute-care hospitals. *Nurse Open, 9*(1), 30-43. https://onlinelibrary.wiley.com/doi/10.1002/nop2.1063
[10] Aimed Alliance. (2024). *Comparing health systems: U.S. and Germany.* https://www.aimedalliance.org

Another difference is fewer German administration jobs in hospitals, as well. Patient satisfaction appears higher, but doesn't that make sense if healthcare is paid for by others? And there is *collaboration* between statutory organizations of payors and providers in creating price caps for certain procedures. Is this possible with competition in a free market? How would this affect the economy? Could this help simplify billing and coding burdens?

All this to say—complex, not simple change will create a tipping point for healthcare reform since America is built on democracy and the notion of capitalism—the American Dream of working hard personally pays off. And other major considerations-- people outside the U.S. are seeking our quality and ready availability of healthcare, our superior research and development, and our ability to choose (See Chapter 6).

Obamacare- As part of the Obama Administration (2009-2016) Affordable Care Act (ACA) of March 2010, the idea was floated of forming a Ministry of Health, similar to Germany, for making decisions. This was a stretch in control by the government—for example, during the Pandemic, might the Ministry decide who should first get a ventilator if there were equipment shortages? You can ponder the implications of that idea. It did not fly.

What did fly in Obamacare was voluntary limited government subsidies for State Medicaid programs, a move to more outpatient procedures (scary but mostly working), and incentives for practices by allowing wellness visits paid by Medicare. The ACA was said to be over 1000 pages in detail for health care reform. Was such detailed implementation at the Federal level even possible, reasonable, and acceptable?

It definitely ramped up the data requirements to tame the beast and drive change. The downside was the additional burden placed on the hospitals with no consistency in information systems and data integrity. In the best-selling book *Search for Excellence*, the phrase data rich and information poor (DRIP) was defined: lots of data but lack of processes needed to produce *meaningful* information, that is essential in creating a competitive business advantage. Maybe this is where the Federal Meaningful Use project was born in an effort to ensure accurate information for trending, then action leading to sustained results. More about this in Chapter 5.

Access - A very important part of Obama's Affordable Care Act (ACA) is presently being threatened. In 2024, increased patient access diminished with the loss of margins and Pandemic recovery. The dilemma: how do you balance access and margin? And can income and expenditure be stabilized?

More hospitals are closing or merging to stay afloat. Some are recovering slowly after losing COVID subsidies. Also, Medicaid subsidies to the states via Obamacare are up for renewal in 2025. Rural hospitals are creating multiple hospital partnerships to decrease supply costs and availability but understand supply costs are only part of the jigsaw puzzle.

In more reform action, Beckers reported (October 2024), four major not-for-profit health systems launched Longitude Health to influence innovative solutions to the industry's biggest challenges. The founding member hospital systems are located across the country: one in Washington state, two in Texas, and one in North Carolina. They will collectively invest for five years, plan to create impact over the first 12 to 24 months, and ask others to join in time. Longitude Health founders believe they will move to change faster at the facility level. This is exactly what my research has revealed. We will watch with interest whether this becomes a turning point for more excellent care, as the influence of these systems has great potential. How will they define "enhancing core operational functions and transformation"? This is great news—American innovation at work.

Chapter 2 TAKEAWAYS

1. Seek the glossary for the many acronyms
2. Obamacare is the accepted step toward fewer uninsured nationally
3. The German model of healthcare has possibilities to consider in the U.S.
4. Access, an important part of Obamacare, is threatened post-pandemic due to mergers, acquisitions, closings, and antitrust focus
5. Innovation at the hospital and system levels is happening to support the margin for the mission while transforming care delivery in pockets

Chapter 3

SIMPLICITY- simplifying the system & cutting red tape

The Health Security Act- standard claim forms for all payors & uniform claims package with standard billing and coding.

A major barrier to direct patient care is paperwork (now mostly digital). The positive goal is to create a user-friendly product but has morphed into software that includes every regulation and dictates how to get there for physicians and staff. It becomes a "check in the box" exercise to assure compliance—if staff either check the box honestly or don't check the box at all. This spurned internal work to drive accuracy in documentation, which is a monumental task globally. You can imagine what Pandemic chaos ensued with agency staff going from hospital to hospital, dealing with various types of electronic records and specific implementation rules for each. This is still causing inefficiencies and delays in patient care.

Years ago, I was asked to implement clinical guidelines for certain procedures, using physician input. It was an impossible task to get the Expert culture to agree. Their overall perspective was a loss of autonomy and decision-making they were trained for and anticipated. Clinical excellence is based on proper assessment, utilization of tests, and timing. This is an art as well as a science. Popular software utilized at this time could be made much more valuable without requiring check box "cookbook" instructions for every patient. It is a dis-satisfier with physicians.

For example, Medication Reconciliation is considered a high-risk, error-prone process—it means every time you visit a health care facility, medication changes made are indicative of an accurate listing when you leave. I know of no known electronic system that supports this well, so the process is manual and laborious, especially with the elderly, who often have a myriad of medications on admission to a hospital. This is a required physician manual task and often is too labor intensive to tackle.

Another example is measuring nurse hourly rounding using the EHR. During the Pandemic, I worked on a medical/surgical unit, partnering with a nurse aide during her shift. We had 18 patients. Healthcare was in chaos and often short-staffed. My partner had to chart every odd hour on every patient that ID band was on, the brake was on the bed, items within reach, etc. The Registered Nurses charted the same list on even hours. Granted, rounding is difficult to measure and an important best practice for safety. However, checking boxes does little to assure patient safety and actually reduces direct patient care time by tying staff to computers at the nursing station.

I know one hospital that has a team to simplify their EHR for clinicians—their initiative will take years as they plow through hundreds of canned care plans. Plans of care are one of the hot topics for accreditors and a top-named deficiency as a deviation from hospital policy. Often, the deficit is a matter of computer documentation versus proper patient care, which is heartening.

Unfortunately, simplification measures were addressed by the Clinton administration but are not evident today, and complexity has continued to increase (Figure 3, Page 46). Simplification is, no doubt, the greatest opportunity to increase employee engagement, decrease turnover, recruit and *increase time with patients*—leading to more consistent patient safety and satisfaction! At one time, Medicare and Medicaid had different data requirements to achieve quality. They finally came together on metrics, so *is that collaboration possible today at any level?*

Last, not least, see Chapter 4 for more on the complexity of billing and possible savings there.

Chapter 3 TAKEAWAYS

1. Paperwork (mainly digital now) is a major barrier to direct patient care.
2. Information systems attempt to police practice rather than be user-efficient and timely
3. Documentation is not adequate to trust the data for improvement
4. Specialty analysts are needed to create reports and are not consistently part of the quality department staff
5. Removing fraud from the industry does not return the value expected and requires large groups of auditors

Chapter 4

SAVINGS- Controlling costs

Health Security Act- Increases competition on price & quality, strengthens buying clout for negotiating contracts.

In 2023 and 2024, the Pandemic pushed resources and finances to the limit. In October 2024, Becker's Hospital Review listed the profit margins for 31 hospitals (not an exhaustive list, but a good representation). Of the 31, only the top 8 margins were over 4%, with 7 at a negative operating margin. Although Obamacare focused on increasing access by assuring rural hospitals remained solvent, COVID uncovered poorly managed and/or underfunded facilities, which then faltered. Now, mergers, acquisitions, divesting, and closing are the actions of the day. Interestingly, the Federal Government is intervening more in mergers and acquisitions, disincentivizing small hospitals and causing more closures out of necessity. Conflicting agendas.

As previously mentioned, purchasing groups are utilized to decrease costs by increasing negotiation clout. In several instances, this cost savings is not enough to keep hospitals open. Economically, wages go up with inflation increasing the inability to recruit to rural areas. Many procedures are moving to outpatient, a less costly venue. However, diagnostic and other equipment required is more and more expensive to maintain and upgrade, while needed for better outcomes and cutting-edge care. Radiology equipment like MRI and CT Scanners continue to take the top spot in the hospital budget, pushing other initiatives aside with no choice but to do so. This is a fact of life in acute care to ensure state-of-the-art diagnostic quality.

I recall Peter Drucker, a renowned business expert, focused on competition being necessary to bring costs down, which translated into changing the way we pay for healthcare. *The Price You Pay* by Dr. Makary[11] explains the pricing game we play at present—certain coding strategies, hospitals pricing high and receiving low reimbursement from Medicare/Medicaid, and cost-shifting to Commercial insurance to cover the cost of bad debt for those who cannot pay.

In creating the Glossary, I am reminded the MOST difficult part of the patient care process is billing. The types of agreements are (and may not be inclusive):

- Fee for Service
- Cost Based Reimbursement
- Value-Based Care
- Professional & Facility fees
- Diagnostic Related Groups
- Global Capitation

[11] Makary, M. M. (2024). *The price we pay: What broke American health care—and how to fix it.* Bloomsbury Publishing.

Ponder how much labor, software, difficult patient processes (and more) would be saved if the billing system is simplified. To address fixing healthcare, this would majorly decrease the money required. And, yes, there are legitimate incidents of fraudulent charging and billing. However, opposed to political opinion, policing the industry by the government has a very high cost with inadequate return on investment. Additionally, hospitals are required by the Department of Justice to have Compliance Programs, focusing on internal auditing of previous and present hot topics provided annually.

Choosing Wisely (Choosingwisely.org) is an initiative created by the American Board of Internal Medicine (ABIM, 2012) to decrease utilization of unnecessary testing. Their goal is to encourage specialty societies to identify—with supporting evidence—which tests, treatments, and procedures are generally needed, and which are not. They report generating many conversations, stimulating journal articles, and inspiring similar campaigns in other countries while improving patient outcomes. This is another demonstration of sharing influence and knowledge across the nation, requiring local hospital input to drive change. Choosing Wisely exemplifies a powerful driver for change with a high chance of notable success, being physician driven.

In 2001, Healthcare Financial Management published numerous articles on healthcare reform. One article describes parallels between manufacturer and health care competition.[12] Both industries experienced increasing market deregulation, changing government policies, and growing consumerism. They concluded that an *integrated* performance-measurement model, as in manufacturing, can help blend hospital strategy with the demands of the environment. Performance-measurement systems drive focus on mission and vision by aligning strategic objectives and resource-allocation decisions with customer requirements (also a Baldrige concept; see Part 3, Chapter 3). Yet, this concept does not often receive investment at the facility level to make it an operational reality. Instead, there is more reliance on the regulator's great quantities of data, which cannot be current, so improvements can be timely and prioritized.

Quality tools and teams are proven means of non-bias problem solving in multidisciplinary groups. Processes become standardized (as possible), and staff pulled to various areas have consistent guidance toward priority goals. I personally observed union and management begin to collaborate on patient care in a small rural hospital using these tools. I sincerely believe this is our operational way forward to strong teams, patient-centered excellence, and—yes—cost control. More on the High Reliability Model (HRO) in Part 3.

---

[12] Stewart, L. J., & Lockamy, A. (2001, December). Improving competitiveness through performance-measurement systems. *Healthcare Financial Management, 55*(12), 46-50. https://pubmed.ncbi.nlm.nih.gov/11765632/

Chapter 4 TAKEAWAYS

1. Mergers and closings are prevalent in 2024, reducing access post-Pandemic
2. At the same time, anti-trust is a renewed focus at the government level
3. Inpatient revenue is diverted to outpatient, lower reimbursement while the cost of state-of-the-art equipment is still required for best quality care
4. The business concept of increased competition decreasing costs is challenging based on the myriads of required community arrangements, making cost accounting data questionable
5. Manufacturing shows Performance-measurement model works to align strategy and allow resource decisions for customer requirements- healthcare lacks the ability to do this accurately

Chapter 5

QUALITY - Making the world's best care better

Health Security Act- increasing consumer knowledge of quality to shop, invests in new research, pays fully for preventive services.

Preventative care is absolutely what all healthcare workers wish for their patients and communities. The reality is many patients are non-compliant and/or have no interest in changing their lifestyles. Although we never give up trying, results are often disappointing and hospital "frequent fliers" exist, utilizing resources without taking personal responsibility. This is their freedom of choice.

CMS and other payors deny payment for some procedures if lesser options are not used first, like Physical Therapy, before booking a knee surgery, which is a good thing. The connection to healthcare benefits for all begs the question: What statistics exist showing whether all people, given benefits for all healthcare, will be good stewards of the gift as fellow travelers pay the bill? At this time, hospitals accumulate bad debt to cover the uninsured, must write off what they cannot collect and attempt to recover losses in other areas. Is there another way?

While preventative care will make us a healthier nation, the systemic changes will take time to affect the next generations. Short-term, costs and effectiveness with the decrease of adverse events must bridge that gap. Harvard's Michael Chernew[13] understands the complexity of that short statement and suggests the answer is not to *increase* resource costs. He and Dr. Makary agree on that.

There is debate on transparency of pricing, allowing consumers to shop. Dr. Makary also addresses the extreme price differences in the industry. Transparency sounds fair, however, unlike a stove or a refrigerator, healthcare costs vary greatly depending on several factors—the most prevalent is variance in physician recruitment and partnership depending on the location and specialties needed.

Also, Critical Access Hospitals with no more than 25 beds are reimbursed by actual costs, while small to large hospitals are now fee-for-service with capped DRGs. The difference in payment was part of the 1997 Balanced Budget Act to assist rural hospitals in servicing residents living a long distance from emergency care. As well, the trend toward outpatient versus inpatient to reduce costs is prudent and may be good for a patient, but not reasonable based on whether there is sufficient support at home.

---

[13] Dafny, L., & Chernew, M. (2024, February 12). *Prevention: U.S. healthcare spending: Myths, facts, & strategies.* Harvard Online.

Data Driven - CMS has, in the last year, pushed for more data from the hospitals that don't have the manpower or the proper systems to glean this data readily. Also, in more and more states, each individual payor has a "quality program" providing financial incentives, some overlapping and utilizing CareCompare (public CMS quality data that lags), and some that do not. For example, Pennsylvania has Highmark, Aetna, Cigna, UPMC, and CMS programs. This requires coordination and more labor to manage the many quality indicators—some of it is relevant everywhere, some not. A recent example is the CMS Health Disparity initiative requiring some parts of the country that are 99% one ethnic group to analyze the 1% to determine whether any nuances can change in their care to increase outcomes. This is non-value added to those communities and increases costs. When inquiring how CMS will measure our success, there was no answer readily available.

The National Roundtable on Health Care Quality was convened by the Institute of Medicine (IOM) in October 1998[14]. This included an "extraordinary assemblage of expertise in the management and study of quality in systems of health care." They found:

1. Healthcare lags behind other sectors in quality improvement- most purchasers do not demand accountability from contracted health plans or providers. They equate quality with the correction of deficiencies rather than continual feedback and improvement of care patterns. They rely on regulators for monitoring and enforcement.
2. Clinical quality improvement efforts, successful in other sectors, must be fully implemented to affect significant change. This requires commitment by top leadership, resources for training and IT support. All stressed the urgency of moving quality improvement out of the special projects area into the mainstream of strategic business initiatives.
3. ***Key Takeaway***: Pressure should be shifted to the *organizational level* to induce changes in institutional performance. Computer technology needs to support real-time clinician research, decision support, and other valuable data for decision-making.
4. Customer demand will increase with aging baby boomers in chronic disease years- they require information and participation in decision-making.

This analysis and resulting Vision resonate fairly well with the 2024 observed reality. However, a follow-up JAMA article published in 2005 stated there was no progress in implementing the changes based on their findings.

---

[14] The Milbank Quarterly. (1998). *The Milbank Quarterly, Volume 76, Number 4.* https://www.milbank.org/quarterly/764featcoye.html

Around the same time the National Roundtable was convened, a small group of Michigan business leaders (home of the auto industry) created the Leapfrog Group[15], starting with simple, focused safety principles to ensure our higher GDP cost was creating positive outcomes: Computerized Physician Order Entry (CPOE), ICU intensivists (specialists on site), and minimum volumes for surgeries determined high-risk procedures. Over 2200 hospitals report voluntarily to their Leapfrog Survey, identifying measures and benchmarks to *leap* to excellence. All benchmarks assist in moving an organization to the next level of excellence, although this is only one data resource of many available and is only available annually.

The original survey is now quite large, the manhours required to collect and submit all measures have increased, and hospitals are questioning the value versus cost due to lower margins. Having been responsible for this survey, I can say there are several sources of data required, and not all data is available from the electronic medical record (accurately), requiring manual collection and coordination.

Then, in 2012, Leapfrog launched the Leapfrog Hospital Safety Grade for all U.S. hospitals (excluding some with small volumes). This is different than the original survey but uses some values to crossover if submitted. Recently, Leapfrog began penalizing hospitals on their safety scores if they are not participating in the large survey by applying a minimal score rather than re-weighting the domain, as in past calculations.

This does not reflect actual performance and is easily misunderstood for public perception and comparisons. The layperson assumption is, for all Safety Scores of A, B, C, D, and F, organizations are measured equally, as it should be. The Safety Grade began as a minimum standard to prove competitive competence across all hospitals but has changed course. At present, limited time and stretched resources at local hospitals need the freedom to adjust resources with specific patient-centered priorities as the main goal—excellent patient care without penalty.

To further clarify, Hospital X participates in the Leapfrog full survey, recording a top score on the Hand Hygiene measurement, which transfers as such onto the public Hospital Safety Grade calculations. Hospital B does *not* participate in the full survey, has top proven compliance in the Hand Hygiene measure but is provided a minimum score instead of an actual score on the safety grade—not comparing apples to apples. This, in turn, affects the total grade. Each year, the safety grade becomes a public relations problem for hospital boards and the reputation in their communities. How do you explain this easily, or is it even an issue in the eyes of the public?

Again, let us beg the question: Does a hospital focus resources based on customer needs and strategic planning for community health, OR focus toward making sure the large

[15] Leapfrog Group. (2024). *History.* https://www.leapfroggroup.org

survey is submitted accurately to Leapfrog every year, protecting public image? Benchmarks are needed and plentiful, but not from all sources—our boards and our community need an accurate source of truth.

As part of cost control, hospitals are also re-evaluating all certifications, registrations, surveys, etc., which provide specific service line benchmarks for excellence. Manual data entry is often needed. So, eliminating this data entry becomes another option to quickly conserve labor, especially with the added data regulatory requirements coming from CMS. More are coming in 2025. But do less benchmarks alerting us of care standards inhibit the pathway to the next level of quality excellence? Some would argue, yes.

The CMS IT (Information Technology) Strategic Plan for 2024 to 2030[16] states well the goal to support consumers and providers with a more complete view of a person's health—meaning a complete and accurate data view. Unfortunately, delivering this goal adds to local data demand at the facility level, aggregated at the Federal level, and published as benchmarking in the form of lagged data. Many organizations are ill-equipped with cumbersome data systems, therefore needing increased labor to comply. This becomes another distraction for adequate, daily patient care. Hard choices must be made on a daily basis to meet data deadlines.

The Federal Government Interoperability Program provides incentive dollars for reaching certain goals in their strategic IT plan. Formally called the Meaningful use Program, Information Systems Departments in healthcare have been achieving specific objectives with electronic health records (EHR) to qualify for incentive payments since 2011. In 2018, the Program's focus on billing-related functions shifted to the exchange of clinical data and increased outcomes and efficiencies, especially at the point of care.[17] A Federal Chief Health Informatics Officer role was created with the noble vision of providing the right care to the right person at the right time more quickly, reducing costs, and increasing outcomes. Again, the analysis and resulting Vision are great, but implementation is slow and inconsistent, burdening facilities strapped for labor—not a criticism, but an observation.

A 2018 article in Healthcare Executive highlights two systems that reached high levels of Interoperability with better billing, reduction of severe harm events, communication between providers, and immediate access to clinical data—while decreasing duplication and reducing costs. Excellent. In 2024 both systems are switching to the same Electronic Health Record (EHR), EPIC, which enjoys over 50% hospital market share now. This is very positive. EPIC is considered the most user-friendly, straightforward and adaptable digital record available. Overwhelmingly, there

---

[16] U.S. Department of Health & Human Services. (2024). *HHS finalizes federal health IT strategy to drive systemic improvements in health and care.* https://www.hhs.gov

[17] Wagner, K. (2024). Interoperability: Success models of digital integration. *Healthcare Executive.*

is agreement EPIC can best meet our need for an integrated, accurate digital view of a patient's health with continued development. The natural selection of EPIC by a market majority will provide a competitive advantage for those utilizing it. The family-owned American company's Vision is that every patient's data should be able to be shared (with permission, of course), wherever that patient goes.

Ironically, EPIC is being sued for monopolizing the IT industry, stealing and blocking competitors—results to be determined. Wouldn't all of us on the same EHR be a GIANT step toward integration? Hopefully, this will provide a step forward if this hurdle is cleared. There are important privacy issues for resolution involved.

Becker's reported EPIC, along with the American Hospital Association and others, asked for revisions of the Federal rule published on August 5, 2024 to define and advance national information system goals. Barriers to acceptance include division over a national patient identifier, information-blocking regulations, and regulations to assure participation in national initiatives. The debate continues while private hospitals and systems continue to choose EPIC, moving toward the same platform in a free market! This demonstrates the Wheatley Theory of Chaos, further explained in Part 2, Chapter 1 - studied proof that a healthy system (general definition) naturally coevolves with its environment by getting rid of barriers to allow a new culture.

NOTE: Leaders, be aware, removing barriers is part of the highest Level 5 Leadership (*Good to Great*) so healthcare can align with the journey to higher reliability. Also included is putting the right people on the bus and connecting teams. More on this concept in Part 3.

EPIC is also connecting to payors directly which decreases prior authorization times, is working on AI support that is user friendly for the hospital setting to detect patient fall risk, and other initiatives. The innovation continues with intent per the founder, Judy Faulkner, who established the company in 1979 from a basement, and maintains a majority market share in a competitive environment.

Chapter 5 TAKEAWAYS

1. Preventive care is necessary, but proof of outcomes takes longer so takes short term implementation and long-term commitment- Obamacare pushed the envelope on this
2. Price transparency does not tell the whole truth (apples to apples)
3. The Interoperability Programs at the Federal level increase labor and decrease productivity if software in specific facilities cannot easily retrieve accurate data
4. Quality improvement needs to move into the mainstream of strategy
5. Pressure should be shifted to the facility level to induce timely changes and allow more natural evolution to excellence – this does not mean more data requests

Chapter 6

CHOICE- Preserving & increasing options

Health Security Act- can follow your doctor into any plan they choose to join, can select from several health plans & option to change annually, makes it easier to live at home than in nursing facilities.

Obamacare Medicaid state subsidy started in the 2021 Affordable Care Act (ACA) and is accepted in 40 states, due to end in 2025. The recent Health Care Affordability Act, introduced in the Senate, aims to permanently extend this and add more states. There are several health plans offered for choice as outlined in Obamacare, and also much variation from state to state in implementation. The caveat for keeping your doctor is if they "choose" to join your health plan.

Becker's Hospital Review, September 25, 2024, reports debate around "repeal and replace" Obamacare has changed to the impending expiration of subsidies. Reforms are not a major focus in political campaigns at this time—a good strategy due to the complexity and difficulty of making promises without a thorough vetting of possibilities. This, however, should not be a barrier to change needed now.

Discussion continues about incentivizing home health care companies, once again—the pendulum swings back as it is reported more home health company rate cuts have occurred in the last 10 years than in any other sector in the Medicare program. The increase appears timely to support this segment of healthcare since most patients prefer home from institutionalization.

Chapter 6 TAKEAWAYS

1. Following your doctor can occur with Obamacare if the doctor chooses to join your plan
2. Medicaid subsidies to 40 states must be extended by Congress for 2025 – it appears to be a priority
3. Home Health discussions are back on the table to incentivize use after rate cuts for the last 10 years
4. In a 2021 report on trends in the uninsured population, 2010-2020 shows a sharp decline since 2010, especially in lower-income populations, but rose between 2016-2019

Chapter 7

RESPONSIBILITY- Making everyone responsible

Health Security Act- Asks drug companies to keep prices down, limits lawyer fees, employees and employers pay something for coverage, with discounts to small business.

First of all, "asking" drug companies seems like a losing proposition ending in inconsistencies. Germany's program *tightly regulates* pharmaceutical companies. This is a major cost issue for America. As mentioned, the present Federal administration decreased the price of insulin, often a big issue for the number of diabetics now and is working on ten more drugs. Adequate insulin is a life/death issue—some patients try to decrease amounts to extend use, a very dangerous practice. So, this is very positive. The entire pharmaceutical industry is undergoing change for more reasonable cost control.

Lawyer fees - Current Pennsylvania law (42 Pa C.S.A 8528) limits damages recoverable against Commonwealth agencies by using a 1978 statutory cap and is even was upheld by the Supreme Court, despite challenges. As a Risk Manager in this state, I observed possibly less frivolous lawsuits, but more research would be needed to compare actual success from state to state. Some healthcare organizations utilize a company that assigns attorneys to cases and holds them accountable for results. This provides more efficiencies for the Risk Manager, including more expertise at hand, learning resources and increased aggregate reporting to provide improvement opportunities.

Shared cost is also part of Germany's healthcare program, managed by the government. As stated earlier, there is a collaborative effort by Federal staff, providers, and payors to decide what is needed. The country's philosophy is solidarity versus capitalism. America has proven very successful in innovation while upholding principles of freedom. Elon Musk is offering to evaluate our deficit—how about a healthcare innovation? The Health Security proposal also suggests a reform NOT run by the government, but with some direction with delivery and cost control in the private market.

Chapter 7 TAKEAWAYS

1. Efforts in government and private sectors are establishing models to decrease pharmaceutical costs
2. This is a major area of concern, but we are reminded of the research/development needs that cannot be set aside for state-of-the-art innovation in disease control
3. The Federal government put a cap on the price of insulin
4. Pennsylvania is a model for research in limiting lawyer fees
5. Agreement is present for reform NOT run by the government, rather, giving direction for delivery and cost control

PART 2

WHAT DO WE NEED NOW?

Hopefully, the overview in Part 1 gave you a general idea of history, time, money spent, and the many players involved in the idea of change management and healthcare reform. Stakeholders include Providers, Insurance Plans, Suppliers, Consumers, Employers and our Government, along with patients. Add to that a capitalistic, free society espousing the American Dream and the various internal agendas outlined. With all that in play, how does a country ensure quality for the 6,129 hospitals in the United States (2023 American Hospital Association)? Further industry breakdown shows the following segments:

Community Hospitals	**5,157**	**Other of Note:**	
Not for Profit	2,978	Rural	1,800
For Profit	1,235	Urban	3,357
State/Local Gov	944	In a System	3,514
Federal Gov Hospitals	**206**		
Psychiatric	**659**		
Other	**107**		

The mere volume of hospitals included in the reform project begs segmentation for a "test of change", a quality term meaning changes are developed within a smaller circle of control before globalizing. I recall a conference years ago showing a roll-out of the Veteran Administration Hospital's new clinical software. It was so futuristic and even graphed vital signs, immediately showing fluctuations over time for real-time clinical use at the bedside, enhancing efficiency of care.

Consider: *Could the Institute of Medicine reconvene the National Roundtable on Health Care Quality from 1998 and tackle a test environment in the 206 hospitals under Federal control?*

In Chapter 5, you will recall the list of that Roundtable's actionable items:

1. Quality Improvement – changing focus from deficiencies to proactive continual improvement tools
2. Strategic shift - Top leadership support, applying resources based on quality priorities rather than strictly on revenues and expansions of service
3. ***KEY TAKEAWAY***: Focus shifted to the organizational level to induce changes in institutional performance (manageable)

4. Information Technology – support research, decision support, and other valuable data for decision-making

Finally, the main takeaway of this book:

The need for expediency in action and support at the organizational level is at critical levels for quality and cost.

Post-Pandemic margins, short staff, retiring baby boomers, and less experienced new staff contribute to this critical perfect storm. Healthcare workers long for a way to work smarter instead of harder, meaning efficiencies must be quick and successful. Many are still recovering from the Pandemic and are still coming out of the Survival Mode mentality. The knowledge base needs protection from further burnout.

Donald Berwick, MD, is a well-known quality guru who co-founded the Institute for Healthcare Improvement and served for a short time as the Administrator for CMS during the Obama Administration. His book, Curing Health Care (1990), strictly confined itself to quality philosophies and tools to drive change.[18] It involved a case study of 21 health care organizations. They learned:

1. Quality Improvement Tools *can* work in healthcare
2. Spending too much time analyzing Processes may slow the pace of change
3. Cross-functional teams are valuable in improving process
4. Getting action is more important than buy-in (also important)

The proven and popular ISO9000 certification manufacturing standards are based on how well all staff perform and can speak to defined processes. I wholeheartedly recommend further study of this certification because I've personally experienced success with their tools, especially process mapping. Process standardization in hospitals, where possible, with specialized processes intentionally applied where necessary, stabilizes patient care and the workforce team. Non-bias, competent quality facilitators assist in bringing process improvement agreement within a team of multidisciplinary subject matter experts. Dr. Berwick, President of the IHI (Institute for Healthcare Improvement), demonstrated success and made us believers, as well as doers, continually proving his point with positive results. This has enhanced the job of quality specialists, allowing them to contribute to and expedite positive cultural change.

So, let's highlight *organizational-level factors* that support the inclusion of strategic quality improvement. This model, in turn, creates a foundation of success where Margin supports the patient care Mission.

[18] Berwick, D. M., Godfrey, A. B., & Roessner, J. (1990). *Curing health care: New strategies for quality improvement.* Jossey-Bass.

CHAPTER 1

Healthcare Industry: Cultural Perspective

Corporate Culture is defined as a combination of values, ethics, vision, behaviors, and work environment. It is the unique blend capable of creating a competitive advantage—meaning an advantage difficult for competitors to replicate, which leads to higher probabilities of success. Of major importance is the ability of top leadership to ensure, during speedy growth, the core culture is nurtured and sustained as changes occur.

Work Environment - Scientist Margaret Wheatley's Theory of Chaos[19] provides a hopeful view, as her research proved (surprisingly) that order that arises naturally, rather than imposed through direction and control, is a very significant path to success. To be healthy, a system must coevolve with its environment. The key learning here is: collaboration, relationships, and team connectivity—simply, get rid of the "power is information" barrier, and a new culture will evolve. She further states, a tipping point in time is necessary for reorganization, though it may seem uncomfortable and out of control. Sounds so simple, though hard to implement. It does suggest an altruistic vision where the entire healthcare team is patient-centered and strong, breaking down operational silos! Is this healthcare's tipping point?

Additional information about actual culture is found in the Employee Engagement Survey, a standard practice in hospitals, every 1 to 3 years. Usually, a chosen vendor provides an anonymous survey, followed by a report segmenting Administration, Physicians, and other Staff. Major accrediting and certification bodies include employee surveys as a requirement to ensure a thorough assessment of the work environment. Addressing gaps and inherent strengths is subsequently used to create a focused plan for building, improving and strengthening the culture. Too often, opportunities identified are not acted upon or do not create remarkable change and better satisfaction. Other priorities may delay or eliminate such activity.

This is unfortunate since employee engagement is defined as a driver for higher patient satisfaction. The premise is, happy employees lead to better, personal patient care. Another known fact—one of the reasons staff seek unions is feeling they cannot change their environment. Something to consider.

Recall in the Introduction, *Leading Transformational Care,* authors submit--*the contentious nature of healthcare is either caused or exacerbated by diverse groups pushing various agendas while actually reaching for the same excellence.* The good news is aligning mutual goals in patient care quality with non-biased multidisciplinary

---

[19] Wheatley, M. J., & Kellner-Rogers, M. (1999). *A simpler way.* Berrett-Koehler Publishing.

facilitation has proven to build teamwork across departments. This facilitation becomes the work of a newly focused Quality Department, along with the usual regulatory compliance and moving metrics to improve patient safety. Changing culture is developed over time, with persistence and commitment.

Medical Schools are re-imagining their curriculums, as well. Because of the increased natural level of student computer competencies, previous barriers in the Expert culture are slowly changing. We can identify more team players (collectives) within the new physician groups; also, some of the older physicians are buying in, and when physicians drive change together, they are unstoppable! Dr. Stephen Kasko, known as a transformational healthcare leader, believes in restructuring medical education to teach humility and compassion, effective communication and empathy. The integration of the science and art of healthcare pulls Experts and Collectives together for the best possible patient, family, and community care.

Vision - The Affordable Care Act (ACA) required an overall community assessment to start as a baseline for action, repeated every three years, to provide evidence of healthy community improvement. A regional committee usually undertakes the project with all stakeholders. For example, when a community discovers their major challenge is a high incidence of stroke, the vision is that all community providers plan together to create solutions as a whole. They use collaboration in determining how best to coordinate care; they connect individual unique strengths, for a smoother patient process and better outcomes. This is opposed to competition for the same customer base, often resulting in duplicating services without appropriate volumes in market share to assure excellence. Examples of partnerships may include education, nutrition, Neurology specialists, access to care, dieticians, and more. It is a long-proven fact performing higher volumes of the same procedure increases the probability of a positive outcome. The Leapfrog group collected data on specific high-risk procedures to further evaluate volumes and outcomes.

Becker's recently reported two rural hospitals, one in Michigan and one in Virginia, have collaborated out of financial necessity. Where they used to compete for the same population, they cannot provide adequate levels of care due to the difficulty of recruiting in rural areas. They are sharing staff to allow patient access and ensure the best outcomes.

FIGURE 2 LEADERSHIP. STAFF & ACCOUNTABILITY

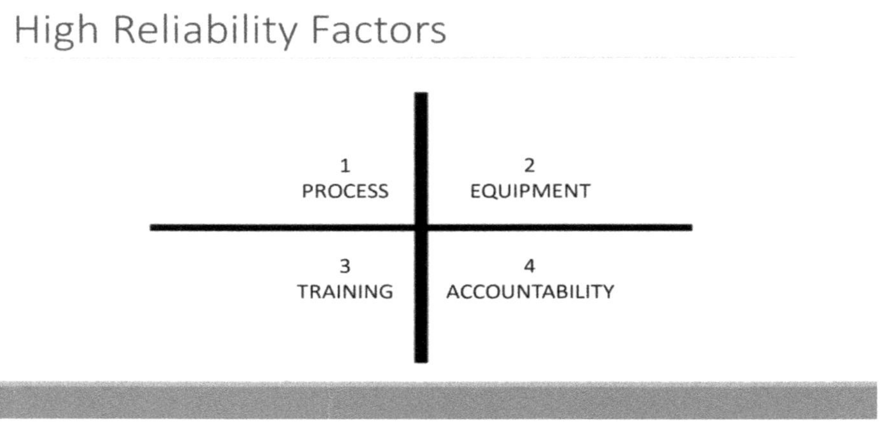

***Behaviors & Values* -** Accountability is a gap voiced in so many organizations when not realizing quality and operational goals. There are many reasons for this, none more difficult than scarce staff. Someone once taught me the following, depicted in Figure 2 above:

Leadership must provide a solid, reliable process, proper equipment, and adequate training; only then can they hold staff accountable.

Of course, managers must follow through with consistent human resource policy, as well. Values are often woven into performance evaluations for annual reviews. However, behavior problems within stated mutually agreed to organizational Values must be addressed as they occur. Otherwise, culture suffers.

This proven process, along with Strategic Planning, creates the highway to reach notable progress in the Vision and Mission of the organization. In Chapter 2, more on how strong Leadership guides Vision, Behaviors, Values, and Work Environment.

CHAPTER 2

Leadership

Vision, Ethics, Values and Behavior factors

A widely accepted leadership concept outlines visionary leadership, positive planning and implementation of change management as essentials for success. The role of successful operations at the management level includes well-designed changes in structure and work processes, effective training, measurement, and reward programs.

I learned about a major leadership resource when starting a business from scratch, called INC., the entrepreneur magazine. INC. emphasized the need for strong, flexible leaders who can change as business grows. The first phase of start-up is called "go-go" where everyone knows you and learns how to team by face-to-face communication while building the foundation. In Phase 2, growth, more people are added, and more formal structures in role definition, policies, and standard practice are communication tools. Different styles are needed for each phase. Even if leaders understand the necessity to transition in their role with the organization, whether they accomplish their own change can mean the difference between stagnation and growth. This is challenging because well-known paths to success may no longer have relevance with growth.

The guru of corporate management, John P. Kotter of Harvard Business School, defines actual transformation as opposed to one charismatic leader causing short term changes:

"In successful transformations, a committed team of leaders and managers guide the effort, but large numbers of people at some time need to play a helpful leadership role in their domain of activities. Only with the combined force of all this leadership can the huge barriers to meaningful change be overcome."[20]

This is a call for leaders with the right skill mix at managerial levels and higher to drive the culture through the business cycle of Start-up, Growth, Shake-out, Maturity and Decline. Kotter also stresses one transitional skill from Phase 1 to Phase 2 is delegation by senior executives, while assuring competencies are adequate in the team to make possible this level of trust. This frees their time for actual strategic leadership. One University hospital where I worked had a policy for top leadership to regularly assess defined leadership skills in their recognized, upcoming leaders, providing a proactive focus on developing a stronger culture over time. What a great retention and investment strategy! Even though Organizational Development exists in many hospitals, I wonder

---

[20] Kotter, J. P. (1996, November). An interview with John P. Kotter. *Quality Digest Magazine*. https://www.qualitydigest.com/nov96/qualview.html

how intentional the process is to identify and connect people, skills, and future strategic planning needs.

Lastly, especially in the service sectors, encouraging the heart is important in assuring engagement. Healthcare draws people who care to give, often pushing themselves too far, at risk of their own health. The caregivers need care. In The Leadership Challenge[21], the authors submit this is possible in three ways:

1. Recognize contributions by showing appreciation for individual excellence
2. Celebrate values and victories by creating a spirit of community
3. Treating challenge as an opportunity
4. My addition – make rounding a priority to show visible support

[21] Kouzes, J. M., & Posner, B. Z. (2001). *The leadership challenge: Encourage the heart (Practice 5, Chapters 10-12, p. 248)*. Jossey-Bass.

CHAPTER 3

Competencies & Development

Recently, I discovered Harvard has a certificate program called Innovations in Teamwork for Health Care. The five-week course claims to "create better teamwork through science." Great opportunity, especially if there are tuition benefits available. I am imaging a whole group with these skills in one hospital which would be amazing!

As mentioned, the Pandemic has caused a steeper learning curve because students were not allowed clinical time to work with actual patients. This means more workload on the hospital preceptors who work with the new staff until competency reaches the appropriate level of care. As the Baby Boomers retire, there are fewer seasoned nurses to precept new ones. Hospital educators are desperately needed to rebuild a strong clinical foundation while assuring regulatory compliance. Too many staff hours are spent at the desk versus with direct patient care. As a CNO, increasing direct patient care hours for staff was a priority and is extremely relevant today. We would evaluate all job duties and determine what was non-value added, or could be delegated or outsourced. The new trend for virtual nurses, added to the onsite team, will be interesting to watch. Will this new role result in fewer adverse events? In the last few years, even before the Pandemic, small hospitals with Intensive Care Units utilized Tele-Medicine to ensure expert availability when a physician is not present. This has worked well to offer support at the right time—I would be interested to hear whether our intensivists who lead the teams would agree.

Historically, a nurse would need some experience in Medical/Surgical care before transferring to higher-risk areas like Intensive Care or Emergency Care. This changed some years ago when another shortage of healthcare personnel required hiring new graduates into critical areas right out of nursing school. Mixed with a shorter two-year Associates Degree Program to become a Registered nurse, and the staff stresses of the Pandemic, the learning curve lengthened. Diploma three-year programs no longer exist, closed or merged with the 4-year programs. In the past, Diploma nurses received a heavy clinical rotation and were known for their ability to hit the ground running upon hire. Fast forward to the need now for nursing internships, residency programs, and preceptors <u>in the hospital</u> to fill the gaps in competencies. Of course, there is a shortage of Master's level nurses to teach in academics as well. If that system returns to full staff, the burden on hospitals may decrease once again. Until then, our Educators are essential in reducing adverse events.

During one stint in a for-profit health system, I was assigned to review and update the competency model. We utilized the Donna Wright model which is still prevalent today.

This involved subject matter experts in each department over 8 hospitals in a room, making changes in the policies using best practices. I developed a sincere appreciation for these leaders who were passionate in their work and ability to improve staff competencies, a big part of patient safety. They used innovation to focus on accountability, empowerment, and ownership versus checklists.

Then, Donna Wright was invited to speak at the Leadership Forum for all 8 hospitals. THAT was very impressive and motivational. I like to tell my friends and family to remember the great clinicians they meet when they are hospitalized—in the midst of the chaos of change, there are competent caregivers who care well and meet individual needs in a safe manner. It means so much for others to express appreciation for their service. We can all "encourage the heart".

CHAPTER 4

Resource Issues

Realistically, hospitals have priorities, and resources are scarce. Facilitation as a skill is also scarce. Because there are so many detours in priorities operationally, I would not begin to judge why. It is unfortunate when opportunities, like employee engagement surveys, are lost to better understand culture from the staff perspective. When input is not recognized, trust and perception of value erodes more with each survey, until people quit talking. A recent Gallup poll, surveying 10,000 U.S. employees in November 2024, found engagement and culture most prominent reasons for leaving a job, followed by work/life balance.

Studies show the drivers of higher costs in U.S. healthcare are: Physician salaries, pharmaceuticals, and administrative expenses[22]. We discussed the work with pharmaceuticals going on presently. In 2018, a Harvard study dispelled an explanation that high costs in healthcare are based mainly on over-utilization. Administrative costs accounted for 8% of total health care spending compared with 1 to 3% for other countries. An employee with tenure shared she observes, over time, the Vice President level builds, then vacates, only to build again in another crisis. I've seen it as well. This then begs the question: are the right leaders with the right competencies in place who can mentor the Director level, decreasing the need for leaders in more levels of care?

The Baldrige Standards for Healthcare outline how resource allocation, a leadership task, ideally begins with Strategic Planning. Only then can leaders project where resources might shift—no longer needed in one area, but more needed in another, and when. Baldrige focuses on a connection between growth, budget, and infrastructure that aligns with the organization's future projections. Asking questions like, for a strong Cancer Care service line growth priority, do we invest in a Nurse Navigator as a new position going forward? At the same time, what service line has decreased in need so the budget can shift neutrally? Can we share physicians and spread out the cost of quality expertise?

I have witnessed planning connected with Strategic Planning in action. That particular system experiences continued success at being one of our most profitable, during and after the Pandemic. Their added advantage is having the transformational team on the same page, making decisions based on the projected Vision. Powerful for maximizing patient care.

---

[22] Feldscher, K. (2018, March 13). Physicians' salaries, cost of pharmaceuticals, and administrative expenses top the list. *Harvard Chan School Communications.* https://news.harvard.edu/gazette/story/2018/03

CHAPTER 5

Incentives

Many hospitals utilize tuition reimbursement to incentivize clinical staff and add to the overall competency of the organization. Some also provide gift cards (or the like) for success in specific areas of patient care for focus, like patient satisfaction. Also, there are Daisy Awards for Nursing, Employee of the Month awards for those who best model values, and Patient Safety Best Catch awards for staff who actually catch an error before it is made. These are just a few rewards and incentives teaming with finance, quality, clinical and ancillary staff when chasing zero harm and its challenges. Incentives are best connected to chosen priorities for the specific organization.

CMS is launching a cohort of three states to participate in the AHEAD model (Advancing All-Payor Health Equity Approaches and Development)—Maryland & Vermont, Connecticut & Hawaii, New York in five downstate counties & Rhode Island. After readying themselves, the kick-off will be in January 2026 or 2027, depending on the cohort. Each participating state may receive up to $12 million for implementation activities over the first 5-6 years. It appears they are promoting the primary care coordination model, which has not thus far gained traction. They are also integrating this with five programs that already exist while taking out two that will overlap. This type of collaboration is hopeful.

The government's AHRQ (Agency for Healthcare Research) launched a National Action Alliance for Patient and Workforce Safety—a collective effort of federal agencies and private partners to improve patient and workforce safety. The goal is a 50% reduction in harm by 2026. It appears voluntary and, like the Leapfrog Group, provides best practice resources. The Dashboard of metrics is substantial—I count 71 different indicators.

It is noted in the Journal of the American Medical Association (December 2005), Physicians Donald Berwick and Lucian Leape stated the problem in healthcare is not bad people, it is the system that needs to be made safer.[23] The AHRQ responded at that time, recommending patient safety surveys at individual hospitals. This is the first step in the 2024 AHRQ safety program, as well.

In 2005, I experienced a definite political clash of agendas over the patient safety survey as hospital administration was wary of projecting an unsafe image of the hospital (reasonable), while more transparency was needed to provide opportunities to improve (also understandable). Many survey questions are open to subjective interpretation—

[23] Five years after "To Err is Human": What have we learned? (2005, May 18). *Journal of the American Medical Association.* http://jama.ama-assn.org/cgi/content/short/293/19/2384

what you think is safe, what the community thinks is safe, and what I think is safe may be different. This becomes a very sensitive public relations subject and may erode community confidence. Can it be successful? I would never say “never” but it would take careful leadership and collaboration. Needless to say, initially, it was discouraged at the facility level, where often the quality/safety group were attempting to spearhead the assessment and action plan development. Conflicting agendas once again.

There are State level associations who provide similar opportunities to advance care from the government side. There are a number of voluntary safety groups to participate in and some choose all, which is very time-consuming because of mandatory regular calls. The other challenge is resourcing since data collection and best practice implementations, overseen by an agency, require actioning and data reporting for accountability and benchmarking. The same labor issue occurs when consultants are brought in to gather data and make recommendations. They must utilize the same staff to gather adequate information for a paid project, then utilize them further to develop action planning and implementation.

This is another reason individual hospitals need leadership to focus on specific Strategic Planning goals, aligning them with specific resources to get them there. Otherwise, we are resource rich and implementation poor, often not adding actual value to the patient.

CHAPTER 6

Information Systems

The Data section of Part 1, Chapter 5, Quality, outlined challenges utilizing present electronic medical records (EMR) for data at the facility and State/Federal levels. The variety of information systems creates differences too extreme to align, working with 6,000 American hospitals. Although continued effort at the government level may get us there, eventually, could the demand for more data be met using a subset of players with the same information system? It is reported EPIC now has market share over 50% of the hospitals and a platform they are piloting with AI for documentation relief. A great sigh of relief may be heard across the nation if our government would consider this. Find something that works, then, as the quality philosophy dictates, spread it across the systems. Tests of change. This could be immediate and far-reaching relief as there are more demands coming from CMS in the pipeline.

One initiative CMS started around 2017 was Electronic clinical quality measures (eCQM), automatically extracted by them from a hospital's EMR. This would take the place of facility abstraction and submission, a grand idea for cost reduction. However, it is now 2024, and though hospitals are required to choose a few indicators from a list each year for CMS extraction, the project is not fully implemented. Abstraction has a big learning curve. As abstractors turnover, hospitals must outsource for high cost or start training again, which has its own disadvantages. CMS also audits local abstraction for accuracy.

Here is the challenge—the electronic medical record has various options for where documentation can reside. CMS extracts the selected eCQMs from every facility into a home base, utilizing the same discreet fields. The number one complaint is inconsistency in staff documentation which can make the difference in passing or failing. And, to be fair, the demands for regulatory and billing documentation are so heavy for staff, it is impossible to monitor and police them all. The advantage to having an abstractor of this information at the facility level is the ability to search and find proper documentation and avoid a deficiency. CMS cannot do this for everyone because of sheer volume. So, although CMS extraction may be a good idea that could reduce costs, the project is still not fully implemented to meet the goal of simplification and efficiency after 7 years in production.

CHAPTER 7

Vulnerabilities

At this point, let us review some of the major challenges in our healthcare crisis based on a clinical and business perspective.

1. Accurate and accessible data for government publication without using valuable resources from patient care at the local level.
2. Building back post-pandemic with a smaller and less competent labor pool due to limited patient care experience during COVID.
3. Push toward more costly preventative mandatory care incentivizing utilization, increasing short-term costs with long-term benefits.
4. Revenue shifts downward as procedures successfully migrate from inpatient to outpatient care while expensive equipment and updates are still needed to provide cutting-edge care.
5. Innovation and the re-evaluation of what additional leadership skills would hasten transition the industry. What experimental trends will work, and what will be harmful? Like virtual nursing?
6. Administrative costs at Federal, State, and local levels exceed those countries with consistent lower GDPs – re-evaluation needed.
7. Competition doesn't work in general for healthcare in the same way it does in most businesses (More in Chapter 8 and Part 3, Chapter 2). There is fear in transparency.
8. Primary Care Physicians make less than specialists and are in short supply with dwindling Medicare payments while looking at a future where Primary Care is the gatekeeper to decrease fragmentation, duplications, and cost with efficiency. Along with this is the need for a pool of competent extenders—Advanced Nurse Practitioners and Physician Assistants.
9. Resources to police fraud do not often supply an adequate return on investment – re-evaluation needed.
10. Baby boomers over 65 are due to flood the industry with more cost, the oldest reaching 84 by 2030, and studies showing most individual healthcare costs occur at the end of life.
11. Information Systems will be key to global connectivity for patients, but local progression must happen as soon as possible – as one author noted, because this is a priority does not mean CIOs have global leadership skills to get us there.
12. Level 5 Leadership as defined in *Good To Great* –Part III Chapter 2.

13. As in all good businesses, SWOT evaluations (strengths, weaknesses, opportunities, threats) analyses require a thorough assessment before final decisions are made as to best paths for the future.

I do not claim to have all the answers. My intent is to provide more input from a clinical perspective to expedite actions by decision makers. Our models of care must evolve quickly to protect our caregivers and patients.

Figure 3 below illustrates stakeholder demands on quality to best visualize healthcare in the present, 2024. It is meant to clarify, not overwhelm. I believe in American innovation and talent—we can and will make it better. We must start at the *facility level* to relieve the burdens and refocus on patient-centered care.

What ideas can you offer for immediate fixes, to start the change conversation where you are? Might regional or service-specific associations influence stakeholders to more intentionally provide the action? Where else might you speak with influencers?

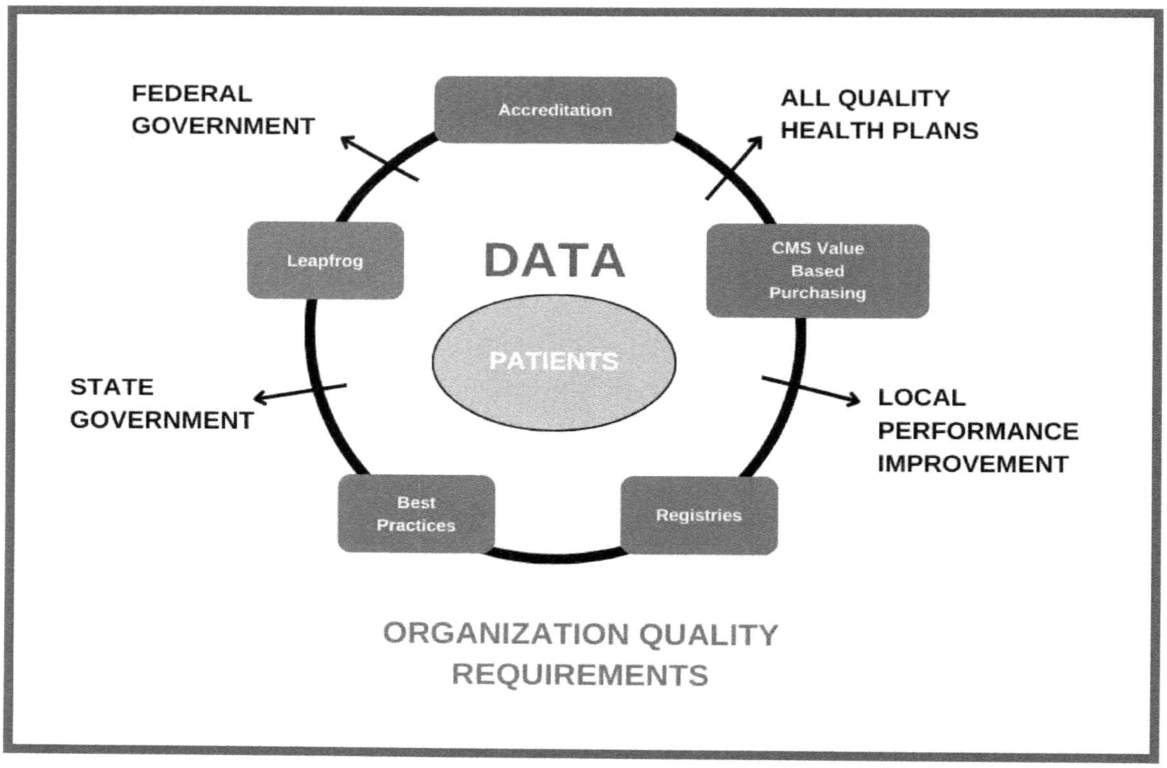

FIGURE 3

CHAPTER 8

Closing the Loop on the HAS

First, I am truly thankful for all the work then and now, in analyzing the American healthcare Industry to assure continual improvement in quality and cost-efficiency. With all the chaos, stresses of the Pandemic, shortages, access issues, and political changes, caregivers continue to make a positive difference. The successes of the last 50 years are amazing—for example, leukemia in children is no longer a death sentence, robotic surgeries decrease trauma and shorten healing times—gall bladder surgery used to be a major undertaking with drains and long hospital stays and now patients return to work in days. Orthopedic surgeries are now performed outside acute care with positive outcomes, decreased chance of infections in-hospital, and fewer revisions over time, an almost expected follow-up in previous years. These are just a few top-of-mind items, but the list is exhaustive. And, the people dedicated to such care are called to a special purpose, to our advantage. As we close the loop on the Health Security Act and look at margin for mission, we remember the people who serve us with thanks.

So where are we? In summary of HAS:

<u>Security – Guaranteeing Comprehensive benefits to all Americans</u>

There remains a philosophical debate that big Government cannot bridge at this time, and evidence that "benefits for all" do not decrease costs.[24] Evaluation of present offerings is on tap with a new administration. There is less push to eliminate all of the Affordable Care Act and look at what works to continue building on a hybrid model, acceptable to the public.

Limiting healthcare premium increases and out-of-pocket expenses is viewed as too much government control and remains a contractual issue with payors for employers. One major barrier is the inconsistency of power to negotiate based on market share, affecting the rural markets and their viability to provide needed access.

Prescription coverage- cost reduction is happening in the free market; more coverage, less out-of-pocket, more expense for somewhere in the economy- cost shifts to be determined.

[24] Prevention: Harvard Online, Feb 12, 2024, webinar, U.S. Healthcare Spending: Myths, Facts & Strategies, Leemore Dafny, Michael Chernew

Expanding Access- at this time, access is decreasing due to low margins and focus on antitrust concerns to maintain competition.

Simplicity- simplifying the system & cutting red tape

In Chapter 3, we outlined many possible payor agreements for which healthcare providers must bill. If we expand Medicaid government subsidies again in the initial 40 states that partook or possibly add more states accepting government subsidies, simplicity becomes more complex. There are too many contracts with too many stipulations negotiated by so many people that benefit pockets of people. This adds to the overall billing costs for providers, acute care, medical practices, outpatient care. And generally, the persons doing the billing may be on a learning curve, since it is very steep. There are many patient complaints about inaccurate bills and/or inability to understand what is billed, even utilizing software programs for this purpose.

Revenue Cycle Management is the process used to manage financial operations starting with the patient appointment, and following with insurance verifications, billing, and collecting, which includes handling denials. This takes a village of people with different skills to get accurate results for services rendered. This process also includes clinical resources which compete with time for direct patient care.

The most extreme example: one large not-for-profit healthcare system implemented a software program, providing daily billing edits to nursing staff showing missing clinical information needed for billing purposes. If the nurse did not correct his/her deficiencies in documentation before leaving at the end of the shift, the manager was accountable for editing them, before she/he left for the day. Although this is an innovative idea, it added complexity. The competing agendas between the Business Office and a burdened clinical staff was highlighted, as they worked to meet all regulatory, patient satisfaction, quality requirements, AND documentation requirements.

This, along with Federal demands for data submission from the local facilities, creates more burden and less time to meet quality goals. Simplicity needed is reduction for staff at the patient level, as soon as possible. Along with billing simplification, data burden is an urgent, major need locally.

Another Vision of the HAS was having health plans focus on more control of quality. This resulted in super-quality programs from various payors that increase the volume of data. Part of my most recent position was to manage all quality requirements in collaboration with our revenue cycle staff and others. Revenue cycle staff agreed they could not be successful without quality driving improvements strategically. The spreadsheet created to analyze commonalities and differences is huge and difficult to manage.

Savings- Controlling Costs

Why doesn't competition work in health care?

Price comparisons for consumers are almost impossible due to multiple types of providers with a variety of salaries at various facilities. For example, a high-level trauma facility (Level 1) requires Neurologists 24/7 as do Comprehensive Stroke Centers, a level above Primary Stroke Centers. How do you compare the costs of a rural hospital that does not provide this level of care with the ones that do? As one business owner with a pending knee surgery stated—"How would I know a deal is a deal to compare?" She shared they don't know how to evaluate even the product preferred for implantation, and there are many. That's what the physicians do well for us.

Some patients who have small out-of-pocket responsibilities and good insurance coverage do not wish to shop and want a healthcare person to guide them—why should they shop if they can ask a provider to refer them to someone they trust to advise them? It's so complicated for the public. Also, it is noted by some that the public will often choose a higher-priced option because they struggle to make a confident quality/cost decision on their own.

This is why part of the German Program for shared cost responsibility is that the young pay for the old, rich pay for the poor, healthy pay for sick, singles pay for families. The responsibility is spread out. There is statutory (mandatory) insurance for those with less of a certain income (considered uninsured), private insurance purchased by those having more earnings and wish for choice, and an employer/employee pool of equal contribution. In the U.S., some citizens may use up savings to pay for a catastrophic illness, while others do not pay but all must be assessed and treated (by law) if they arrive within so many feet of the Emergency Room doors. One CEO made the point that this does not happen in any other business.

Small hospitals may provide better access but are unable to negotiate prices with health plans—no purchasing power. Lately, this has resulted in a number of hospitals reducing services, like Maternal Health, a low margin service line but desired by communities. Also, the cost of cutting-edge diagnostic equipment is prohibitive and often a barrier to entry for newer or smaller facilities.

Finally, and I am sure others could cite more reasons, the competition in healthcare begets fragmented care. When I visit an Internist, the provider refers me to specialists for everything (my experience). Versus a Primary Care Provider who may biopsy a mole in the office rather than send a routine procedure to a Dermatologist (higher cost specialty care). Physicians are incentivized to refer to each other for their specialty—yes, the care is higher level and, granted, needed many times but sometimes not.

Choosing Wisely is an example of how dedicated physicians push to decrease unnecessary utilization of resources. This expands focus for all resources—providers, lab, imaging, equipment, revenue cycle, etc.—on the areas of need. If successful in changing the culture, this effort will increase efficiency exponentially.

The final chapters in this book will address *Good to Great: Social Sector* by Jim Collins. It is a very intelligent approach, also expanding the profit motive. That is, collaborating with quality and disciplined operations creates momentum that fixes margin. This resonates with so much we have discussed.

Quality- Making the world's best care better

In The Health Security Act, opening up knowledge for consumers to price care when purchasing healthcare is thought to increase quality by "shopping". As we discussed in Chapter 4, competition in healthcare is not so straightforward for deciding the best deal.

Preventative Care will no doubt increase our national health by better controlling the root causes of chronic illness but will take years to realize. So, what can we do for increased quality excellence in parallel with prevention work? Dr. Chassis, the previous president of the Joint Commission on the Accreditation of Hospitals, made the case that *consistent, high reliability* is needed. Also, many organizations began using the principles of a High-Reliability Organization (HRO) to further progress. In all my travels, I observed examples of what this could problem solve, especially with staff being pulled to other units or contracted labor dropping in and out. The more efficient and consistent processes are, the less chaos exists for the patient and the staff. In fact, Part 3 explains this Vision in more detail.

Measurement against an external benchmark is a Baldrige requirement. More on this challenge and reality in the last chapters, as well. Bottom line—we must have some measurement to aspire to or mediocrity will ensue. When our local organizations only look at internal improvements, they may be getting better but not performing anywhere near the rest of the U.S. hospitals. CMS CareCompare does assist in benchmarking, but data is lagged by a quarter and aggregated for 12 months at a time, making more agile and timely changes difficult.

Interestingly, a 2018 Harvard publication on health care costs also reported the quality of care once people are sick is high in the United States.[25]

[25] Harvard Chan School Communications. (2018, March 13). *Health care costs: Physician salaries, pharmaceuticals, and administrative expenses top the list.* https://news.harvard.edu/gazette/story/2018/03

Choice – Preserving & Increasing Options

Following a doctor into any plan only works when the doctor chooses to join your plan—or you move to one in which they are participating. There is an opinion the Obamacare plan choices are a legitimate compromise to Universal Healthcare and further reform might be built on this piece. Researching the advantages and disadvantages is beyond the scope of this publication. However, I am sure we will see more debate on this in the near future.

Home healthcare incentives are back after a long time when increases in the industry to keep up with inflation were not adequate. This forced divestiture by many owners. There will likely be an increase in service again.

Until more of the government "fixes" are implemented, working on what can be done at present must remain the focus here.

Responsibility- Making everyone responsible

For those not wishing for Universal Healthcare as a solution, there is agreement that reform should not be *run* by the government; rather, they should stick to *delivery and cost controls*, for example. Public opinion is more and more costs are transferred to patients via increased deductibles and out-of-pocket increases right now. And, these are often surprises at the time of care that are very different than past coverages.

Discussions will commence on shared responsibility mechanisms for adequate money to support healthcare as reform is further defined. American cultural norms are unique when compared to others. Customers (patients and families) require short waiting times, choice, proper billing systems, knowledgeable clinicians, state-of-the-art equipment and ready access to care.

All we know right now is our healthcare costs exceed others by about 6% of GDP. Those drivers are medicines, specialty physicians, nurses, extenders, administration and competition for the same services. Salaries differ in the U.S. mainly because we recognize the risks of less education and want to afford more opportunity. Germany's nurses are reported not to have specialty training so more burden is on the provider!

There are many role duplications between payors, hospital staff, and physician offices that annoy and confuse at times. While a patient, I used my physician office nurse as my "go to", my insurance company was calling me with a case manager (which I declined), and hospitals were providing comprehensive cancer care, along with hospitalists, if admitted to hospital, outside of my surgeon and oncologist. While I had excellent care, I recognized my advantage in navigating my care because of more knowledge of how the system works. Coordination of care decreases costs overall and treats the patient to more efficient care—trips to the hospital, extra imaging and bloodwork, and more referrals to more specialists that could be handled at a lower level of care.

Researchers agree there is no easy fix. Discussions will include where we are willing and/or must pay based on our nation's public requirements for excellence. Is a shared responsibility model, as in Germany, possible in the U.S. with any modifications to balance all of this?

PART 3

PRINCIPLES FOR STARTING & BUILDING TOWARD VISION

CHAPTER 1

Vision

In 2016, Dr. Peter Pronovost, a quality physician and Director from Johns Hopkins

FIGURE 4 HIGH RELIABILITY JOURNEY

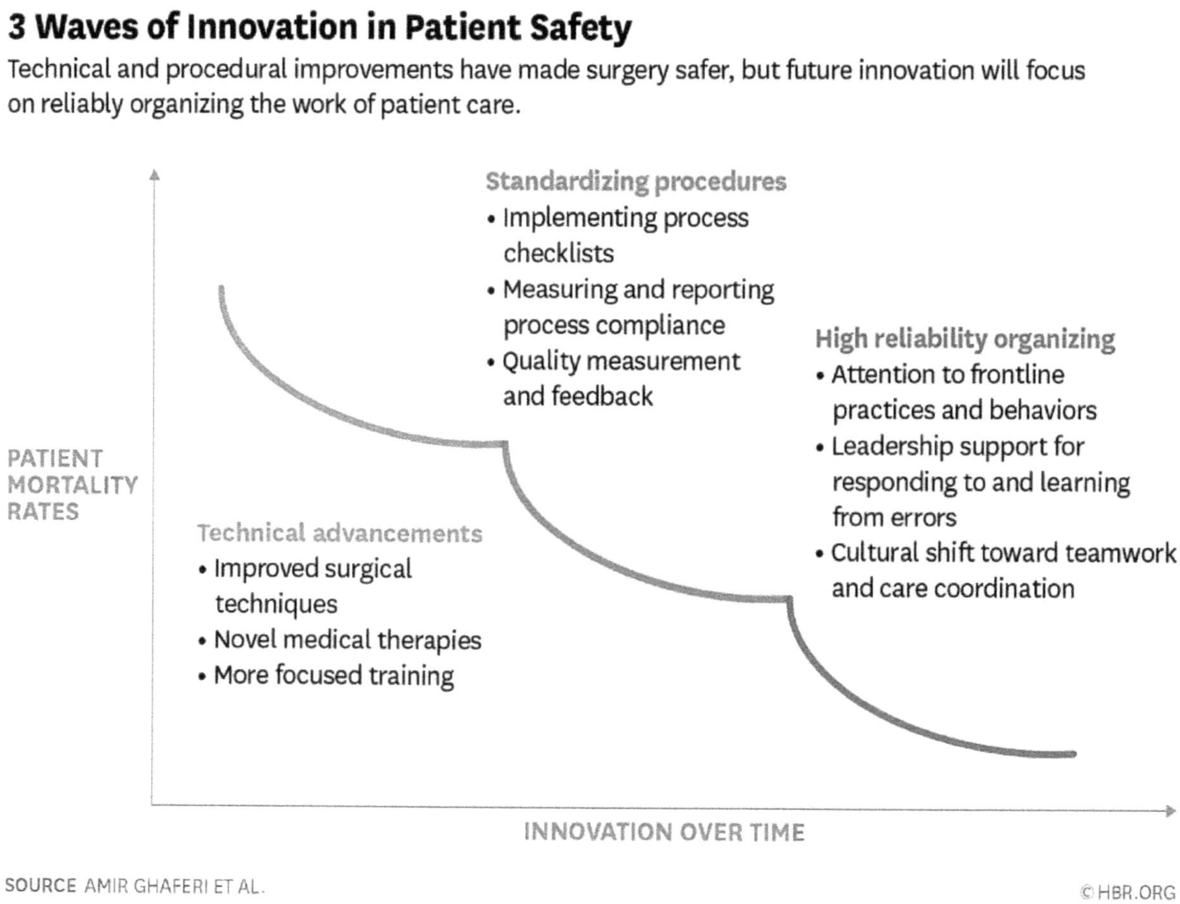

Medicine, co-authored a piece in Harvard Review outlining what needs to happen in the next wave of increasing patient safety.[26] It is called High Reliability and he claims, for higher performance, we must deal with how people interact and organize their day-to-day work. They realize over-standardizing increases risks, so balancing standardizing and embracing variation is needed. Here is their visual:

[26] Ghaferi, A., Myers, C., Sutcliffe, K., & Provost, P. (2016, August 8). The next wave of hospital innovation to make patients safer. *Harvard Business Review*. https://hbr.org/2016/08/the-next-wave-of-hospital-innovation-to-make-patients-safer

In Part 1, Chapter 4, titled Savings, we pointed to quality tools and teams for providing resources and multi-disciplinary team facilitation. This includes reviewing processes, standardizing where possible, and allowing intentional variation as needed.

In Part 2, Chapter 8, titled Closing the Loop on the Health Security Act, we discussed the original 2011 article republished in 2017 from the previous President of The Joint Commission making the same case. Upon assignment in a hospital Quality Department, I seized the opportunity to present these reputably based theories to Boards, Providers, Senior Teams and other Leaders. Afterward, I facilitated teams for higher reliable processes—it caught on very well with various leaders requesting process reviews in many service areas, as well as trying process mapping on their own! Consistency of patient readiness for surgery before arriving at the surgery suite was one example of a successful collaboration, using the tools. This improvement led to decrease in surgical delays which led to cost savings and surgeon/staff satisfaction.

Let me expand on the Dr. Chassis 2011 article, published as a guide to developing high reliability in healthcare.[27] He describes, historically, attempts to improve clinical quality over the last fifty years have met with limited success. Examples include increased competition, public reporting, re-engineering, and total quality management tools like Root Cause Analysis and Failure Mode Effects Analysis. We still have pockets of excellence at individual hospitals or on specific measures, but these efforts are not consistent and often not sustained.

Where are we today? For the calendar year 2023, there were 1411 sentinel events (serious) reported voluntarily to The Joint Commission. Falls, wrong surgery, delays in treatment, and unintended retention of a foreign object remain in the top five bad events. These are listed every year at some level despite all the work to prevent them. Failures in communications, teamwork and inconsistent policy use were the leading causes the Joint Commission cited.

High-Reliability Science is utilized in Commercial Air Travel, Nuclear Power industry and Flight Decks on aircraft carriers to maintain extremely high levels of safety. A common key feature identified in achieving this level of excellence is a collective mindfulness—everyone is aware that small failures in process can lead to catastrophic outcomes.

How does healthcare get there?

- Leadership long-term commitment- includes Board, senior managers, physicians
- Safety Culture- staff trust, report, and see improvements in safety

---

[27] Chassin, M. R., & Loeb, J. M. (2011). The ongoing quality improvement journey: Next stop, high reliability. *Health Affairs, 30*(4), 559-568.

- Robust Process Improvement- switching from purely reactive to adding proactive approaches to eliminate risk, using performance improvement tools (non-bias) as shown in Figure 5, below.

FIGURE 5 CONTINUOUS IMPROVEMENT CYCLE

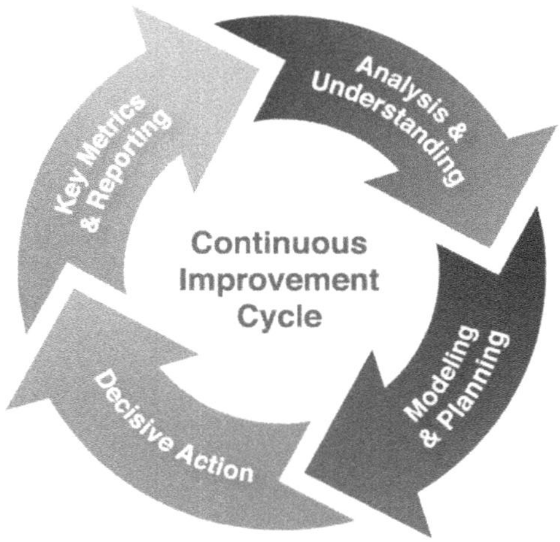

He concludes by recommending hospitals assess their Stage of Maturity in each requirement, using the model:

- ✓ Minimal maturity – focus only on regulatory actions needed
- ✓ Developing maturity – CEO leads *proactive* quality agenda
- ✓ Approaching – *organizational* proficiency in ROBUST process improvement

The Institute for Healthcare Improvement education expands on the main principles needed to define a Highly Reliable Organization (HRO):

- Sensitivity to Operations- good understanding of the current situation; take concerns of staff seriously and elicit feedback
- Preoccupation with Failure- address any level of technical, human or process failure (reaction)
- Deference to Expertise- value expertise over authority in high-risk situations for rapid response
- Reluctance to Simplify- challenge long-held beliefs and use data, benchmarks, performance metrics
- Commitment to Resilience- the ability to anticipate and improvise for the unexpected, allowing quick recovery

They further comment **the path is still clear and viable in healthcare despite the complexities in the industry.** There are many organizations adopting this model, implementing it with a personal touch for their organizational culture, including the military. Accepting the move toward high reliability's migration (See Figure 4, Page 54) offers a more stable and organized patient experience, increasing trust wherever patient care happens. The model is universal--the size of the organization does not matter. *Leadership matters*.

For a visual of the possible new Vision utilizing what different, proven models that exist, see Figure 8, Page 69.

The next chapter provides information on another great source of proven business acumen. We will discuss more about how both of these models intersect for greatness. Then, in the last chapter, we overlay similarities and how the changes may result in the highest American quality award, the Baldrige National Quality Excellence Award.

CHAPTER 2

Good to Great- Social Sector Wisdom

Good to Great[28], published in 2001, has had a profound impact on the business world. Jim Collins and team conducted an in-depth analysis of 28 companies showing 15 years of low performance in the stock market, followed by a clear and sustained transition to high performance for at least 14 years. This credible study allowed them to identify common specific factors separating *good* companies from those who take the leap and become *great*. Because of its enduring value using credible research, it is a must-read for anyone driving organizational success.

In 2005, he published a follow-up monograph for the Social Sectors, extending the concepts and identifying similarities and differences.[29] His passion for learning and teaching in social sectors, adding to discussions with over 100 leaders in education, healthcare, government, and not-for-profits, drove him to produce possible customized applications. He suggests both books must be read together to understand the sector, even stating his team found concepts of the original book valid for healthcare: Level 5 Leadership, Diversification, and Discipline.

Particular questions cropping up repeatedly by social sector leaders are synthesized into five issues, forming the framework for success:

1. Defining "great"—calibrating success without business metrics
2. Level 5 Leadership – getting things done within a diffuse power structure
3. First Who – getting the right people on the bus
4. Hedgehog Concept – rethinking an economic engine without a primary profit motive
5. Turning the Flywheel – building momentum by building the brand

Social sector or not, the Collins team extrapolates from research that greatness is, first and foremost, a function of conscious discipline. This underscores the need to choose and *not* choose growth and services rather than duplicate what already exists, best utilizing scarce resources. Mediocre service duplication offers no competitive advantage to boost margin for fulfilling mission, actually diluting it. The major challenge for collaboration in patient care is smoothing the transition between services in a different location, ensuring a seamless continuation of care. Of course, a competitive market is always an underlying hurdle to negotiate.

---

[28] Collins, J. (2001). *Good to great: Why some companies make the leap and others don't.* Harper Business.
[29] Collins, J. (2005). *Good to great and the social sectors.* Harper Business.

Defining Great in Healthcare

The quality question makes this interesting in the social sector. If volumes for procedures or services are high and more profitable than local competitors, how can quality outcomes be assured and measured comparatively? It is difficult to ascertain whether mortality rates or readmission rates are the best measurements of outcomes with all other factors, but presently what we have to compare. This year, CMS added a new outcome measure -- patient surveys upon initial hip and knee procedure with resurveys for the same patients after one year. However, differences in populations and policies skew comparisons. Hospital X may choose to take on higher-risk patients, while Hospital Y may limit high-risk procedures, making mortality rates as outcomes appear better overall. Because communities differ and always will, specific organizations must analyze their own results, identifying outliers to justify differences internally and externally. Depending on the information systems in place, the hours used to prove or disprove outcomes may be substantial. Could this time be better used elsewhere?

A team in one hospital verified, after years of struggle, focus on improving quality inputs rather than auditing outliers improved quality metrics (required by its highest volume payor's quality program). By inputs we mean efficiencies in process, like turnaround times, standardizing, and accountabilities, leading to more positive outcomes. Revenue Cycle (Finance) and Quality collaborated, agreed and worked together for the overall success: Quality + Finance = Operation Efficiencies & Increased Quality.

Author Collin's example of a social sector redefining "great" is The Cleveland Orchestra. Facing deficits exceeding 10%, a small, stagnant endowment and a struggling local economy, the leaders were interviewing for a new executive director. When asked by a candidate what they wanted to see him do there, the Board replied, "Make an already great orchestra even greater, defined by artistic excellence". *How effectively we deliver on the mission and make a distinct impact on communities relative to resources is the better focus for the social sector*. This is visually shown in Figure 7 (Page 64), where the Hedgehog Concept is discussed

A relatively unknown dichotomy involves regulatory rules protecting healthcare organizations from disclosing details discussed in the quality improvement realm. This often conflicts with the public's need to know "why" things happen and what we do about them. The intent of the regulatory protection is to provide staff a safe place for transparency within the organization's quality forums, prompting more open, focused action for future prevention. This honest explanation satisfies the majority of patients and families. However, without a proper explanation, the perception is sometimes misconstrued as hiding something. Hospitals are committed to a robust system of reviews to glean proper information in reaching for patient safety and cause/effect. A customized annual quality improvement plan is required for hospitals to participate in the Medicare and Medicaid Programs. And, most State regulators hold hospitals accountable for errors.

Additionally, hospital unit leadership has a separate obligation to implement a just culture format in coaching, discipline, or termination, depending on employee performance. Quality sticks to assuring a higher reliability process, allowing management and human resources specialists to provide accountability for error. Effective care meetings with families also develop a relationship of trust to continue using the hospital in their community for their personal care.

Level 5 Leadership in Healthcare

Collins found that Social Sector Leadership has a higher level of difficulty due to complex governance structures. As in government, healthcare has multiple stakeholders with no overall executive authority. The type of leadership required includes a special skillset for empowering and holding accountable various players in their specific venues. With this skillset, the Vision is successfully achieved and with excellence. As John Kotter was quoted in Part 1, Chapter 2 — "...only with the combined force of all (players in) this leadership can the huge barriers to meaningful change be overcome."

Collins hypothesizes there are two types of leadership—one in most pure business circles that allows "executive" style leaders to succeed. While in the Social Sector, skills required are more "legislative". The latter relies more on persuasion, political relationships, and shared interests for the right decisions. Level 5 leaders (versus Level 4) are ambitious first for the cause and work involved instead of themselves. It is not about being nice or inclusive or consensus-building. They make sure the right decisions happen, no matter how difficult or painful, for the long-term greatness and achievement of the mission. He theorizes that, most likely, they require a blend of executive and legislative skills.

Collins Key point: "True leadership only exists if people follow when they have the freedom not to."

Level 5 Leadership in the Social Sector requires an attitude of professional respect for team member capabilities andtheir unique contributions toward the greater good. It raises the level of daily management to visionary leadership. The next generation of youth hails from the digital era of infinitely available knowledge and is truly without comparison to previous generations. Just the thought of many mini-leaders pushing toward the same Vision is inspiring.

The projections of what staff really want from an employer support this leadership development at many levels to strengthen the foundation of a hospital. I shared how one organization identified potential emerging leaders, then planned development over time to retain and build stability.

Another tool used successfully is the 9 Box Grid (Figure 6 below), allowing for a thorough analysis and intentional action planning for experiences to increase knowledge, taking into consideration personal readiness. Personal investment and communication, by including staff in future plans, increase loyalty and retention. This action also addresses the vulnerability of staff turnover, which is so prevalent in healthcare.

Additionally, there may be a positive effect on deterring staff from seeking union support. Follow-up on engagement feedback has already been mentioned as a stabilizing factor, as well.

FIGURE 6

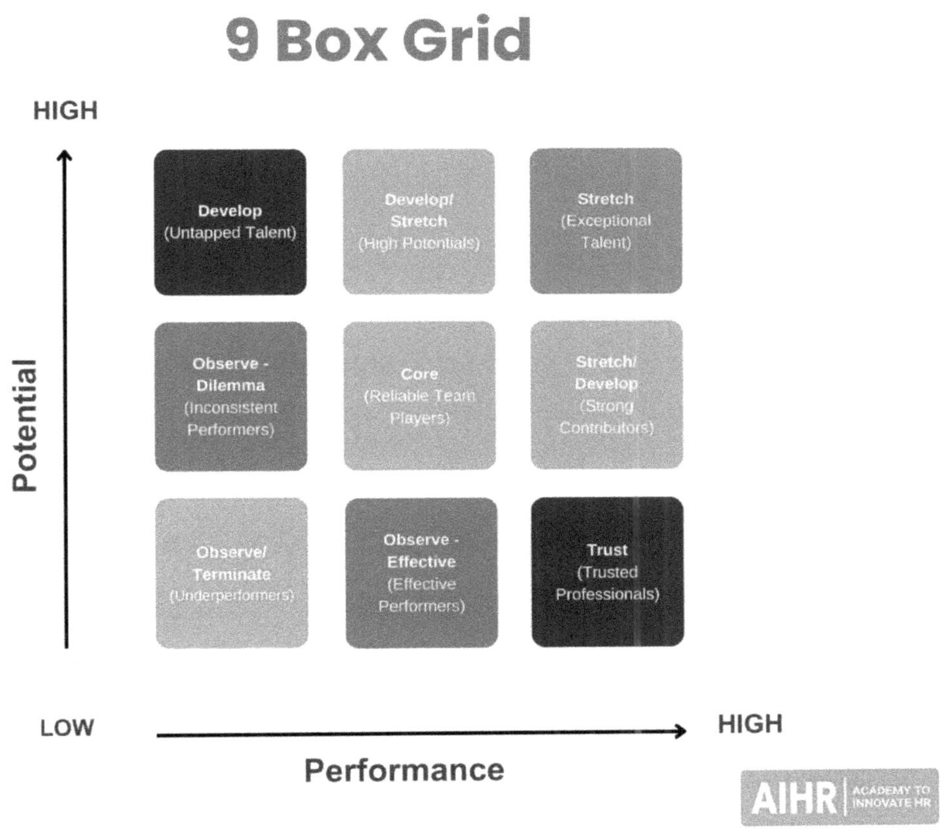

The question has been raised whether a leader experienced in a profit sector business can translate to success in a healthcare organization. It really depends on the person, the leaders involved, and the readiness of the organization. The more directive, decisive style must be balanced with the persuasion and relationship-building of the stakeholder groups involved. We discussed the importance of physician partnering as a way of creating a collaborative relationship with more of the Expert group.

Lastly, a leadership discussion would not be complete without discussing the how and when of personal coaching. The Vision of the best Leadership team possible involves meeting with learners where they are during crucial career-building moments and inspiring change. In Napa, they taught me the best wine was made from grapes that withstood a weather challenge that year. I would submit change is painful, and with the right support at critical junctures, the learning curve can actually be expedited. To this end, I plan to be part of that process as a coach and hope others will consider this to hasten the build toward a stronger, stabilizing future.

One last thought—coaching is not counseling, and sometimes both are needed at the same time. Counseling is a more in-depth analysis with a trained therapist to resolve past barriers. Coaching is rather a partnership to push the envelope of thought, apply new intentions, and become all we are uniquely meant to be in the life domains of Career, Social, Financial, Physical, Community, and Physical. One organization assigned an Executive Coach to each of their C-Suite Leaders during their orientation who continued their partnership as they normalized their roles within the group. As Leaders, offering that support, along with the usual Employee Assistance Programs at crucial times, would be of great benefit for home and career.

Getting the Right People on the Bus

The Collins team point out, for the social sector, reliance must often rely on people underpaid relative to the business sector. Therefore, great companies focus on hiring and keeping the right people. It is a lengthy and difficult process to remove the wrong person, so front-end selectivity is vital. A major key is to focus on self-motivated and self-disciplined candidates who passionately do the best they can no matter what—it is in their DNA. Interviewing well can determine this. Some hospitals use standardized testing, which may or may not add an advantage.

In his book, author Collins provides various examples of how the “right people” focus assisted the leap to greatness. In healthcare, the tendency is to promote excellent clinicians into totally uncharted managerial and leadership positions. Although deserving due to past performance, often an additional skill set is required creating a risk they are not the right fit for the bus. So, approaching hiring differently, takes rigorous attention to the actual job description duties, and intentionally evaluating candidates by using them in a customized interview process.

How, then, does one manage staff feelings of rejection and resistance while repositioning the infrastructure with as little disruption as possible? By leadership promoting consistency in a more selective process, and believing with this strategy a position becomes more attractive. Also, planning for *communication and buy-in* as part of the change management process. The right people also attract other right people. All this supports the premise that increased employee engagement stabilizes culture, improving recruitment, loyalty, retention, patient safety and resources to sustain the mission (revenue).

Leadership must be strong enough to make hard decisions, stress personal development in an actionable manner, and communicate the Vision in a way that touches passion and commitment to safe patient care.

<u>The Hedgehog Concept[30]</u>

This section of *Good to Great* brings it all together. Author Collins has analyzed the nuances of the Social Sector, which resonate strongly with the redesigned healthcare Vision we seek. In addition to their defined Steps 1 through 3 (metrics, Leadership, people), the movement to great requires a series of good decisions made consistently on the three parts of Step 4, the Hedgehog Concept (Figure 7, Page 64). These parts must be well executed, and accumulate one on another over a long period. They found that companies that did *not* leap to greatness tended never to clarify and exhibited inconsistency with scattered behaviors. Consistency in leadership is SO important.

Why is it called the Hedgehog Concept? Isaiah Berlin divided the world into hedgehogs and foxes based on the Greek parable, "The fox knows many things, but the hedgehog knows one big thing".

The essence of this Concept is piercing clarity about how to produce the best long-term results and relentless discipline to say no to the opportunities that fail the hedgehog test. I have witnessed so many times the chaos ensuing when each opportunity is re-evaluated based only on what is happening in the short-term; often due to urgent need for cash flow. In healthcare, the pendulum swings from clinical focus to financial focus in an extreme fashion. The following is an alternative, though it takes bravery.

---

[30]Collins, J. (n.d.). *Concepts: The Hedgehog Concept.*

Here is a visual of the Hedgehog Concept:

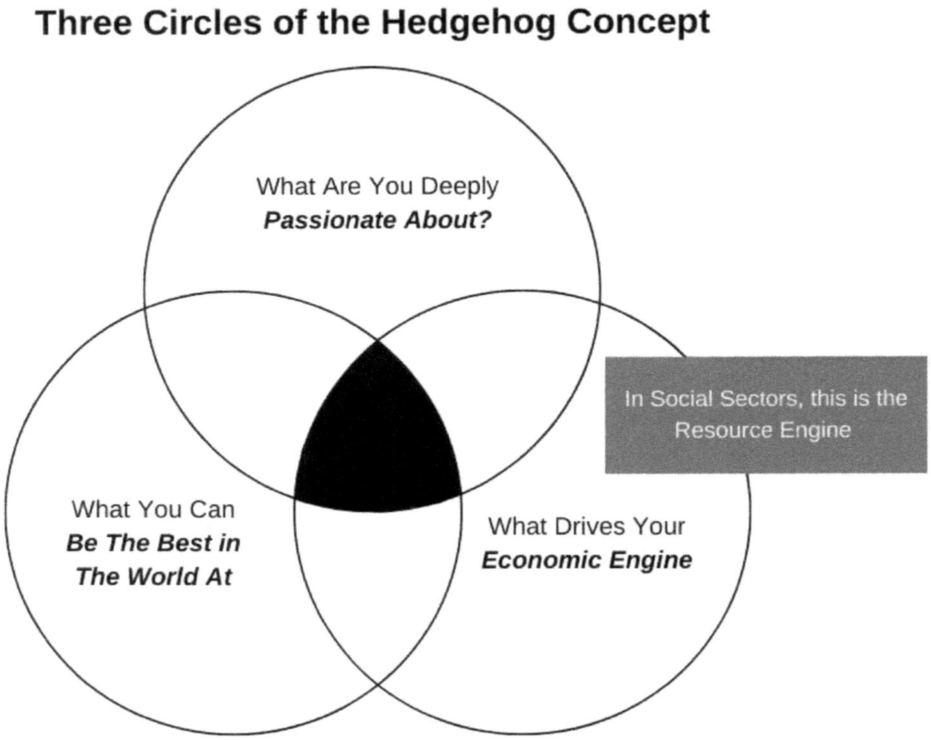

FIGURE 7

The following is the explanation for the **Social Sector**.

Circle 1: Passion = Core values and why the organization exists (mission or core purpose)

Circle 2: Best at = how can we uniquely contribute to patients better than any other organization on the planet (Core Competence).

Circle 3: Resource Engine- understanding what best drives it in terms of time, money, and brand

Research additionally revealed the many types of not-for-profit companies in the social sector, explaining the differences in operations and challenges. They concluded healthcare most closely resembles that of a for-profit business.

The critical analysis is how all circles connect to support each other. Or, "How does focusing on what we can do best tie directly to our resource engine, and how does our resource engine directly reinforce what we do best?" This involves defining what the organization's specific competitive advantage is and leveraging it at critical moments to avoid diluting the entire mission. Much food for thought.

Turning the Flywheel

Here is the beauty of *Good to Great* in healthcare. All those "right" people on the bus start pushing in the same direction. When people begin to see results, they get excited to contribute and want to become part of the momentum, energizing the turn of the Flywheel. In the past, a lack of focus on the Hedgehog Concept led to what healthcare workers call "the flavor of the day". Turnover has become the norm including more and more changes, which then forces the goal to survival, replacing the push toward excellence. Part of my job as an interim consultant was to quickly assess the big picture and recommend what was needed to balance cost and quality showing positive results to move the flywheel. The patterns were often the same. Leadership was challenged to chart a solid course to the Vision, build trust with results, and retain talent to stabilize the organization over time.

Another challenge to success lies in cultural norms of power and competition, as pointed out in Part 2, Chapter 1. We see pockets of excellence in collaboration and partnerships. I would like to converse with many subject matter experts on the Collins Hedgehog Concept to establish innovative ideas for rapid change resulting in a healthier healthcare future. On top of the many plans already in motion, we have mentioned, there is much more. How do we push the national flywheel? And/or start a groundswell of purpose in the midst of a competitive marketplace? I believe in the American intelligence and innovation to do so if we come together.

"American business and industry are beginning to understand that poor quality costs companies as much as 20 percent of sales and revenues nationally, and that improved quality of goods and services goes hand in hand with improved productivity, lower costs, and increased profitability."

-- Public Law 100-107, August 20, 1987
Macolm Baldrige Quality Improvement Act

"America's economic strength depends on industry's ability to improve productivity and quality and to remain on the cutting edge of technology. And that's why the Malcolm Baldrige National Quality Award is so important."

-- President Ronald Reagan

"You must be able to answer the question, "How does focusing on what we can do best tie directly to our resource engine, and how does our resource engine directly reinforce what we can do best?"

-- Hedgehog Concept, *Good to Great and the Social Sectors*, Jim Collins

CHAPTER 3

Baldrige: National Quality Excellence

The Malcom Baldrige National Quality Award was established by Congress during the Reagan administration and named as a tribute to his Secretary of Commerce Malcom Baldrige, who died in a rodeo accident. The goal was to address the Asian and European auto manufacturers who were besting American companies in competitiveness. In 1999, its scope expanded to healthcare and education. In 2007, nonprofit/government organizations were added.

The Baldrige Performance Excellence Program (managed by the Federal National Institute of Standards & Technology, NIST) offers a pathway to connectivity and, based on rigorous standards and site surveys, rewards organizations demonstrating high-performance alignment with sustained outcomes. It continues as an annual Federal award for excellence, awarded by the President of the United States or a delegate. State awards for excellence, based on the same standards, must be obtained before applying for the Federal award.

Having the opportunity to be on the Board of Examiners was a deeply intellectual experience. Teams of examiners are grouped from all over the U.S. and assigned an application to analyze based success in meeting the standards. Examiners come from various occupations and educational backgrounds. This diverse think tank requires hours of debate, ending in consensus and scoring to compare applicants. The top-scoring organizations are then scheduled for site visits by the Baldrige Board before making the final decisions on recipient awards. I have had the honor to participate at the State level in 2 states and 3 times at the national level. I also authored the initial Texas State Award for Performance Excellence application for a system that subsequently won that award, so I can speak for the rigorous process that proving success entails.

This award, with its standards, reinforces the connectivity between several critical systems identified in the standards. It begins with Strategic Planning, and asks for organizations to demonstrate, with evidence, how communications, customer relationships, compliance, workforce, comparative data and performance measurement align to produce sustained results over time. Points are scored for approach and deployment (implementation).

What I learned was exactly what the Collins team discovered in their intensive studies they call the Hedgehog Concept. Both Baldrige and the Hedgehog Concept stress the actual ability to deploy and get results that last over a sustained period, using connectivity. Winning the State level, then the National level can take an average of 5 years and is named the "Baldrige Journey". The NIST website states, "For more than 32 years, the Baldrige Excellence Framework® has empowered organizations to accomplish their missions, improve results, and become more competitive." It is a most impressive endeavor with obvious improvements in organizations that win the coveted award.

I was fortunate to work with an 8 hospital system in a specific regional location. There were 30 teams, and with consultant assistance, we trained grassroots leaders and staff to implement improvements at the same time in all the hospitals, standardizing as we were able. I loved that job! It fed my passion to improve patient care wherever I landed, and together, we succeeded.

When working as a quality consultant, part of my initial organizational assessment was to determine where they were in their quality journey. Leadership could then decide where to start improvements, based on their readiness and ability to commit. Then we could select a specific choice of quality improvement models and tools for next steps based on the organization's maturational level. All three models presented, High Reliability, Good to Great, and Baldrige, are possible pathways to next levels of excellence. Accreditation standards also provide a starting point. I also realized an organization can utilize the Baldrige concepts without committing excessive resources to the actual journey, therefore preparing for future application.

Discipline of purpose, dedication to community needs, and the requirements of patients and the workforce combine to push the Fly Wheel toward greatness. *Good to Great and the Social Sector* describes a great social sector organization as one with the discipline to attract and channel resources at their defined core and to reject resources that drive them away, making it "*...of greater service to the world.*" Well said!

FINAL WORDS

The last three chapters present research pointing to healthcare's need to think differently and intentionally about all parts of the *Good to Great* findings. Let us ask--what is possible for each stakeholder segment to change in their corner of the world in the next 3 months, with more actions in the next 6, 9, and 12 months? I would submit to those whose goals support Universal Healthcare or Benefits for All as a final Vision, we need your collaboration for first steps toward smoothing present processes to offer a more solid healthcare experience to all.

Figure 8 below visually depicts a possible building strategy toward excellence, using the High Reliability, Good to Great, and Baldrige criteria to guide it.

FIGURE 8

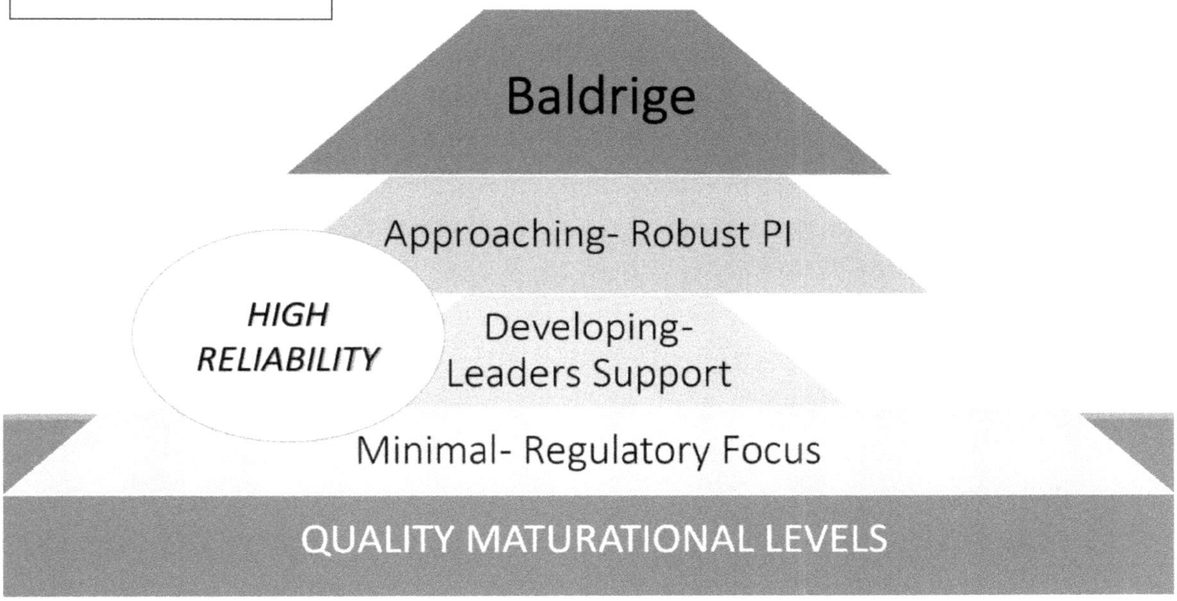

While many wonderful private sector changes are occurring with the innovation of major players, coordinated deployment is missing in many sectors. For the year 2025, we highlighted the CMS AHEAD program, Cuban's Cost Plus, Longitude Health, Choosing Wisely, much of Harvard's work in the Public Health arena, and the AHRQ Safety initiative, to name a few. All of this is very positive and encouraging.

For so many years, the primary focus has been on fraud, which, granted, has some merit based on evidence. But it has not been and is not the silver bullet to decreasing costs and making quality better. This is evidence of how focusing on our resource engine in the social sector requires pivoting dollars away from more auditors. Consider using proactive process improvement along with the usual reactive work (when mistakes happen) to simplify processes, improve patient safety and reduce the ability to commit fraud. I will end with my thoughts on summarizing, based on our analyses, suggestions to consider for each stakeholder group.

Positive Food for Thought

Federal Government

- Incentivize to increase Primary Care Providers who coordinate care
- Simplify ICD10 Codes (complexity increased from ICD9)
- Consider patient access needs with evaluation of antitrust – continue to incentivize physicians fulfilling roles in rural, low-access areas
- Reconvene the National Roundtable on Health Care Quality -- create an action plan to stimulate higher reliability and develop how best to deploy and move the organizational local levels to high reliability- consider tests of change
- Immediately re-evaluate what data is appropriately required by 6000 hospitals, what is needed to address the imbalance, and return our care to the bedside by decreasing data burden. This includes, as Baldrige outlines, defining customer and workforce requirements to support those decisions.
- Evaluate competition and resource engine needs – move past price transparency in a process too complex to compare and move toward what we can standardize for simplicity since variability is known to increase error
- Focus on long-term goals of decreasing chronic disease, while evaluating now how to improve nutrition, agriculture and other inputs
- Assure the right people are employed on the Federal and State regulatory bodies- evaluate all administrative costs and focus resources in the right places for the quality mission
- Find a way to allow the sharing of patient information, requiring EHR vendors to collaborate if competition can be re-examined – this is a major roadblock and very costly

STATE GOVERNMENT

- Collaborate with regional providers to map access and quality needs- consider each focusing on strengths to support what they do best
- Evaluate whether the right people are on the bus for the future Vision
- Work with local organizations whose quality metrics are not up to standards to evaluate leadership and operational gaps for success
- Mandate or incentivize (or both) Leadership standards and accountabilities
- Regulate state-controlled Medicaid
- Incentivize and work with education to increase consistency in provider extender competency
- Aggregate data and take responsibility for state-wide improvements based on benchmarks
- Partner with the Institute of Healthcare Improvement to customize deployment strategies

HEALTH PLANS

- Standardize and simplify billing, prior authorization, and payment
- Incentivize quality and better define measures within their populations- utilize existing data or assist local organizations in specific requirements based on their vendors
- Consider navigator assistance in areas of need
- Stop duplicating case management for patients; very confusing and not coordinated – coordinate with primary care providers and other community providers; determine best patient-centered resolution possible

HOSPITALS

- Assess the entire staff for organizational development opportunity for potential leaders and deploy actions toward meeting those needs; aim for exemplary, strong existing and succession leadership to assure Level 5 performance end in mind
- Evaluate the work environment with the selected Employee Engagement tool, follow through on fully understanding results, and create mutual goals toward strengthening financial and quality sustainability
- Reassess the value of certificates, registries, and Leapfrog surveys against labor costs, turnover, and best practice results
- Provide resources for new nurses with developing competencies, including Educators and assure them ready-access for questions in critical situations (Example: ICU Telehealth where an intensivist can be utilized when a local intensivist is not on site or not available).

- Formalize and structure processes proactively, as possible, using performance improvement tools and staff to provide non-bias facilitation and assure progress- allow for building of facilitation skills
- Assure Human Resource metrics are included, like time to fill vacancies, turnover, and percentage of vacancies, to maximize efficiencies and problem-solve with evidence when barriers occur
- Negotiate wisely for Health Plans, using defined workforce requirements for employee retention – control the Wellness initiatives to collaborate with primary care providers
- Routinely partner with providers on standardization of product choices and monitor, escalating efforts if not reasonably successful
- Provide navigators for cancer patients or where care is fragmented between specialists with little Primary Care coordination

CONSUMERS

- Speak to Unit Leadership first when a problem arises- escalate concerns to supervisor, next level up from direct caregivers, and or quality department; A patient satisfaction coordinator or a team of leaders may assist with difficult resolutions.
- Know your patient rights and hold organizations to those rights
- Always communicate with staff if you are not trusting your environment for any reason
- Tell staff when you appreciate their excellence and attentive care
- Work with a Primary Care Provider for coordination of care

In conclusion, thank you for your passion for safe healthcare and for reviewing this book to seek more understanding. 2025 has the promise of change and movement in Healthcare Reform. Even with multiple priorities, each caregiver is highly aware we all need and deserve the best practices possible. You can trust the wonderful clinicians out there, proven when the Pandemic caused critical survival pressures in the environment around them. I believe healthcare is great in the U.S. Can we do better? Yes, always!

Please join me in the push for more quality excellence. We have shown healthcare is not a partisan industry. Better coordination, collaboration, and partnerships are within our grasp.

Each of us makes a difference wherever we are.

www.ingramcontent.com/pod-product-compliance
Lightning Source LLC
LaVergne TN
LVHW070857210926
848482LV00016B/956
9798349349485